THE ART *of*

Joyful

ACHIEVING

Tapping Into a Life You Love

THE ART *of*

Joyful

ACHIEVING

Tapping Into a Life You Love

JOE MITCHELL, ESQ.

To the Reader

May You Achieve Your Big Goals and Say "Wow"!

As you read this book, I have some additional resources to make your experience even more powerful. You can access them for free at:

http://www.activateyourgreatness.com/joyful

Please make a moment to access and download these now - they will be helpful as you read.

Table of Contents

Praise for *The Art of Joyful Achieving*

Engaging and insightful—this book shows how success and happiness can go hand-in-hand!

— Marci Shimoff,
New York Times **Best-Selling Author of** *Happy For No Reason* **and** *Chicken Soup for the Woman's Soul*

Bringing boundless energy and enthusiasm to helping people transform, Joe Mitchell has provided a step-by-step system to use powerful mindset techniques to achieve your goals. If you're looking for specific tapping scripts to remove your block to achievement this book is helpful!

— Pamela Bruner
Co-Author, *Tapping into Ultimate Success*

For so many of us, reaching for life's big goals is fraught with stress and worry. In *The Art of Joyful Achieving*, Joe Mitchell shows us another way. He combines time-tested motivational approaches with tapping, an acupressure-based stress reduction method validated in over 100 scientific studies. He clearly explains how to find the most compelling vision for your life, and then release the habits and beliefs that keep you from achieving it. His personal story, of learning to stand up for himself as a child, then becoming in turn an attorney, a monk, and a coach, is a demonstration of the power of a clear vision. Yet it also illustrates that we all evolve through different stages; these principles are essential in each new phase of our lives. Anyone seeking a clear path of action to living a visionary life will find this book packed with wise advice and essential tools.

— Dawson Church,
Award-winning author of *Mind to Matter* **and** *Bliss Brain*

Tapping can be a profound ally in moving towards your desired goals, and this book gives you strategies to use it more effectively. If you want to achieve greater success - and do so more joyfully - this book is a powerful guide."

— **Brad Yates**
tapwithbrad.com

The keys to creating the results you want in your life and work are all within the pages of this book. Pure gold. Put aside everything else you're doing and dive deep into these practices. The sooner you do, the sooner you will achieve anything you set your heart to.

— **Fabienne Fredrickson,**
founder of *Boldheart.com* and author of
Embrace Your Magnificence: Get out of your own way
and live a richer, fuller, more abundant life

Joe Mitchell's book The Art of Joyful Achieving is a well written guide on how to create systems and use powerful self-development tools to help you create the success you desire.

In this book Mitchell outlines his own 6 DARING steps success system and challenges the reader to go for it. Many of the usual important elements are there, including finding your why, breaking your goal into achievable steps, developing action plans... but the secret sauce in this success recipe is adding the acceleration power of tapping.

Tapping has proven benefits in relieving stress and anxiety and is one of the most exciting additions to a peak performance plan for releasing inner emotional blocks that can impede performance. In his book Mitchell outlines the steps for using tapping in a straightforward manner then gives us some ways to make the process more accessible and user-friendly. He also gives plenty of helpful examples that the reader can follow to apply tapping to their own success blocks, to free up energy and power for success. He then focuses in on 3 common success blocks that he sees that hold people up, tolerations, procrastination, and lack of self-confidence, and offers helpful strategies for getting on top of these issues.

Of course, taking action is where most people come unstuck and this is where Mitchell draws the reader towards his key message: Planning is important, and action is essential, but actions must be meaningful, and both action and achievement can be and should be much more joyful. The key, and this is where Joe's book shines, is learning how to apply techniques like tapping to make the process more stress-free and enjoyable, establishing what he calls a joyful action routine. After all if you don't enjoy the journey then perhaps you don't really succeed.

Joe gives plenty of pointers to help us step forward in the direction of joyful achievement and I believe his book will help many to progress down that path.

— **Steve Wells,**
Psychologist and Peak Performance Consultant,
Author of *100% YES!*

If you're ready to follow a clear path for success, you've come to the right place. Joe Mitchell's "The Art of Joyful Achieving" provides high performance strategies to help you release your limiting beliefs and up-level your success with joy. It's time to be empowered, and Joe offers the roadmap, the tools, and the support to help you release your blocks and reach your goals with passion and precision. Enjoy!

— **Carol Look,**
Founding EFT Master Author,
Attracting Abundance with EFT
www.CarolLook.com

Joe Mitchell offers an enthusiastic and beautiful roadmap for raising your vibration and transforming your life.

— **Michael Bernard Beckwith**
Founder & Spiritual Director, Agape International Spiritual Center
Author, *Life Visioning and Spiritual Liberation*

Acknowledgments

I WANT TO thank a number of people who made a real difference in my being able to get this book into your hands:

I am very appreciative of those who helped me organize and edit this book: especially my book coach, Michelle Vandepas, and my book editor Shauna Hardy. They kept me on the straight and narrow and helped me to organize my thoughts into a useful book.

Many thanks to Founding EFT Master, Carol Look, for her contributions to some of the tapping variations mentioned in the book such as Thank You Tapping, What If Tapping, and Argument Tapping. Also deep thanks to Steve Wells, the creator of Simple Energy Techniques, Provocative Energy Techniques and Intention Tapping who has had a big influence on my creation of Freestyle Tapping. And a huge shout out for my other remarkable mentors in the tapping world, Dawson Church, Pamela Bruner, Brad Yates, Margaret Lynch Raniere and Gene Monterastelli. Finally my gratitude to Fabienne Fredrickson, Kiva Schuler and all the wonderful participants in the Boldheart Business Program for their ongoing support and encouragement while I wrote and refined this book.

Introduction

Stepping Up

"**H**ELL NO—I AM not going to stay back. I refuse!"

Even as an 8-year-old child, I wasn't going to settle. My African American family had just moved from an inner-city ghetto neighborhood in Boston to an all-white suburb in the early 1960s. My teacher had just told me that I should repeat second grade because the all-black school I had come from was not up to speed—I told her no.

I stood firmly and I never looked back. Yes, at first, getting good grades was a lot harder than when I was in the ghetto school. I needed extra support from my family and my teachers. But by my second year, this little black boy was doing great and in sixth grade he went into his first honors class. Even though I was the only black kid in my junior high school, I was also the only black kid on the honor roll at my junior high school.

From that early time onward, my life has been all about stepping up: going from inner-city schools and almost being held back, to enjoying the scholarly achievements of graduating from Stanford University as an undergrad, and then proceeding to get my law degree at Harvard Law School. I started playing tennis competitively when I was 13 and became the number one player on my high school tennis team, helping our school to win the New England High School Championships during my senior year.

A little later in life, stepping up meant having the guts to leave a promising legal career to follow a deeper passion: studying with my spiritual teacher as a monk for five years. And later, when I chose to return to traditional life, stepping up meant starting my own law practice while deeply focusing on my spiritual and personal development. I learned to be proficient at criminal and personal injury law as a sole practitioner through pulling myself up with my own diligent studies and practice. Now, in this current period of my life, stepping up means embracing the process of becoming a respected coach, speaker, and trainer. And even when I have mastered my new career, there will always be another level to which I will aspire.

What I have learned in my 60+ years on the planet is that the life of a successful person is consistently about stepping up and growing. There is never a time when you have completely made it—regardless of your financial status or the amount of fame or comfort you have gained. To be genuinely successful means that you consistently enjoy your life now and that you have things that you are looking forward to. Even more, it's never finished; I call it **the joy of ongoing self-development!** Are you up for that?

What I Want You to Get Out of Reading This Book

I wrote this book because I want to empower you to create a life of both success and fulfillment. Moreover, I want to help you get clear about your big goals and why you want them. And I want you to create an effective strategy to get to where you really want to go with a smile on your face. But to actually make your dreams happen, I am going to focus our work together on helping you release your limiting beliefs about yourself. I will teach you the DARING Success System, which is a step-by-step process designed to get you past your self-imposed limits and to move you powerfully toward your dreams and goals. By the end of this book, you will have integrated the clarity, mindset, and strategy to:

- Get excited about and envision yourself achieving big exciting goals or anything you want for that matter

- Get clear on your next significant step in an important life area

- Develop an identity for yourself where you are the kind of person that joyfully achieves (without ongoing overwhelm and stress)

- Activate your Powerful Why as the daily fuel for moving closer to both your long and short-term goals

- Release any habit of procrastinating on important things

- Stop tolerating below average and negative behaviors from yourself

- Incorporate great work strategies to move towards your goals quicker than ever before

- Believe and then know that you can create a life of abundance, impact, and satisfaction

This book will focus on empowering you via an amazing tool called tapping. Tapping has worked magic for me, and it will for you as well. By learning the simple process of tapping on certain meridian points on your body, you will be able to move beyond the places where you have been stuck in the past and to supercharge your intentions for success. The DARING Success System integrates tapping with clarity and high-performance strategies that you can apply to achieve the big juicy goals that you will set for yourself.

You will also learn how tapping can help you to create a new identity for yourself as a Joyful Achiever. You will come to know that you can habitually amplify the feelings of joy, confidence, and openness as you take your steps forward. I believe that with the right approach and intention, any one of us can be a Joyful Achiever who dares to make great things happen in our lives and in the lives of others.

The tools and support laid out in this book and the accompanying materials are a reliable system to surpass the struggles of your past and make big things happen in your life with joy. What I want you to bring to the table is the desire to live a life you love and the determination to test drive tapping and the other tools, tactics, and strategies outlined in this book. My desire is for you to discover (or reaffirm) that there is an awesome way to live that is within your grasp. And, even though you shouldn't expect yourself to do it perfectly, you can expect to create a juicy, exhilarating, and fulfilling life for yourself. Perhaps more than anything, I wrote this book to help you have that.

Chapter 1

Achieve Big Goals with Joy... Be DARING!

"All serious daring starts from within."

—*Eudora Welty*

A S YOU READ this book, I dare you to realize that not only can you accomplish the big juicy goals that maybe you've hesitated to even try for—but that you can also achieve them with a smile on your face. Sounds like a pipe dream, right? Maybe you gave up on going for big juicy goals a while back—well, stop it! It's time to get back up on the horse! I invite you to learn the DARING Success System and do some work with the awesome transforming tool called tapping that powers it up. Tapping is one of the most powerful personal development techniques available today. I call my version of the technique Freestyle Tapping, because with the way I show you how to tap, you have maximum freedom to do it just the way you want to. When you combine freestyle tapping with a few affirmations and visualizations, you can very quickly create a feeling of success.

Before we dive into the details, let's first take a big-picture look at the DARING System. Each letter stands for an important practice for Joyful Achievers wanting to achieve big goals.

D - Decide on your Wow Goal

As you begin to direct your thinking to what you really want in your life, I will ask you to keep this word in mind: Wow! Think about your goals by asking yourself these questions: What goals, if I accomplished them within the next year, would bring a feeling of Wow to my life? Please think big! And then consider why accomplishing these goals excite you. Feel the Wow! You will choose one of these Wow goals which we will use to implement the DARING Success System into your life.

A - Activate the Power of Tapping

Activating the Power of Tapping will allow you to release your negative emotional blocks and increase your motivation. We will learn and explore both traditional EFT (Emotional Freedom Techniques) and Freestyle Tapping (my version of the process) that enable you to quickly let go of the negative feelings of stress, anxiety, and fear as well as the limiting beliefs that have held you back from being your best self. Once the unwanted mental and emotional junk is released through what I call "Release Tapping", you will move on to affirm your power to joyfully achieve your Wow Goal with "Power Tapping".

R - Release the Big Three Limits to High Level Success

Limiting beliefs are a key reason why you don't already have what you want in life. Many of us have unknowingly created a glass ceiling that keeps us from moving higher. A large number of would-be high achievers are stunted in their progress by what I refer to as the Big Three Limits to High Level Success: tolerations, procrastination, and lack of self-confidence. This step is all about identifying and releasing your particular blocks in these areas, even if you can't completely articulate them. This is an utterly important step in claiming your power and allowing yourself to move forward with ease. You can also use this process to release the blocks that you are experiencing in any area of your life.

I - Install Your Joyful Achiever Identity

Your identity (who you say you are), controls your results. If you are hesitating, by changing your identity to be a confident and unstoppable person, you will massively change your results. In this step, we incorporate joy as a powerful ingredient that makes achievement more fun and less of a hustle and grind. You are going to learn how to quickly turn on your Joyful Achiever Identity, so you will be able to create this empowered joyful state whenever you get off track.

N - Nail Your Meaningful Action Plan and Get Started

Next, we are going to discuss how to consistently take meaningful action and create a solid plan that identifies powerful strategies and tactics to achieve your Wow Goal. You'll learn to make the journey to your Wow Goal into a prioritized and actionable plan and we will start to help you integrate the Joyful Achiever Routine into your daily habits. And when you do feel stress, you'll have your tapping tools and a few other smart strategies to help get you right back into a stress-free state. The goal is for you to feel passionate and unstoppable as you take small but meaningful steps forward.

G - Get Support

Now that you've empowered yourself and you have a plan that you are beginning to implement, it's time to get support to keep you on track. The benefits of getting an accountability buddy, being a part of a mastermind group, hiring a coach and working with a mentor are discussed in detail here. It is important that you don't feel like you need to go at it alone—the truth is that there is great support out there for you as you move toward 'Wow'!

I hope that your curiosity has been stimulated by this brief introduction to the DARING Success System. Before we dive in more deeply, let's do a quick exercise. Cup your dominant hand into the shape of a 'C' and place the pads of your fingertips right below your collarbone. Start a firm, gentle, and regular tapping rhythm. Keep the tapping going as you affirm the following sentences. The most powerful way to do this is to say the sentences aloud with conviction. If you want extra credit, say them three times! Even if you are not entirely ready to embody these affirmations right now, do your best to say the words like you mean them:

I am ready to take my life to the next level with joy! I am willing to let go of anything that has held me back up until now as I see and feel the new awesome me. I am becoming more skilled at shifting my emotions and appreciating myself. I believe I can do great things because I am willing to be DARING.

Then smile (even if it's completely forced!) as you keep tapping. Perfect! Put your hand down and take a deep breath. Now... congratulate yourself! Really acknowledge yourself for doing this exercise. You have just taken the first step on your success journey and I want you to realize that there is power in acknowledging even your smallest wins.

Chapter 2

D - Decide on a Wow Goal

Dream Big and Say "Wow"!

"The biggest adventure you can take is to live the life of your dreams"

—*Oprah Winfrey*

YOUR AMAZING LIFE starts with clarity and focus. What do you want to achieve? What desire excites you so much that when you think of achieving it, all you can say is "Wow!" That's your first DARING task: to create a long-term vision and a short-term mission that wows you. Choose a big objective that you really care about. And let's get started...

Get Enlivened by Your Life Vision

Let's begin by creating a compelling 360-degree vision for your life and then intentionally getting excited about it. You don't want to get too busy sprinting to accomplish stuff (even if it seems meaningful) until you connect with where you want to go in the long run—the big goals and accomplishments that will make you go "Wow!" three to ten years from now. You could be a little frustrated and regretful at the end of your life if you waste a lot of time running up a less-than-fulfilling hill (even though you might look great running up it!). It's time to get clear on your Big Juicy Long Term Goals and know why you want them—this is known as your Life Vision.

Your Life Vision is composed of clearly stated big intentions in the major areas of your life. The beautiful thing is that youcan most likely accomplish your Life Vision if you take consistent action and pursue it in the long run with dedication and determination. You will likely need to break out of your comfort zone again and again and act even when you are feeling afraid. But the good news is that taking consistent small steps towards a clear and inspiring vision can lead you to big opportunities and, eventually, to major success.

Creating a compelling vision for your life is one of the major purposes of a well-known personal development course called Lifebook, which is run by Jon and Missy Butcher. When I completed the course a number of years ago, we dedicated four full days to creating a picture of our ideal life in 12 different life arenas. By the end of the four days we had created a very special book, called our Lifebook, which contained our hopes and dreams for our lives on Earth. It was one of the most valuable projects I have undertaken, and almost ten years later, I still go back and revisit my visions for the different areas of my life.

Let's now do a short but powerful exercise designed to help you define your best life. Review each of the following life categories as you think clearly about what you would love to experience. As you define, get clear on, and imagine accomplishing your desires in each of these areas, make sure that you envision an accomplishment (or two) that makes you exclaim "Wow". While we are primarily focusing on outward achievements and worldly goals in our discussions throughout this book, it is my intention that you create and pursue a "Wow" vision in each of the five major life categories below:

1. **Health and Vitality:** This category comes first because without your health in at least decent shape, life is difficult and not a lot of fun. Taking care of your physical self is a critical job and those who do it well are rewarded with zest, vitality, and energy. There are major opportunities in the times we are now living in for the average person to be physically vital and thriving, even at an advanced age. This category is controlled in large part by the fundamentals of diet, exercise, sleep, and stress-relief, so make sure you have all of them nailed. As you think about your health and vitality now and in the future, what would be a "Wow" for you to create?

2. **Relationships and Love:** This category is what activates your heart energy. The relationships in your life are also the framework for your service to the world. Take a few moments and envision creating powerful, loving, and fulfilling relationships with your significant other (or, if you don't currently have one, finding that special someone), and your family and friends.

3. **Career and Finances:** This category is about your contribution and your legacy: it's the area where you will probably spend the most time and make the most differ-

ence. How can you create your career in a way that you love? Your finances are an important focus too—achieving big success in this area can lead to an amazing sense of freedom and excitement.

4. **Spirituality:** This category is about your relationship with God, the Divine, or a Higher Power. What is your vision of an ideal relationship with the Almighty and your expression of spirituality in your daily life? Do you dream of unconditional love, peace, or divine grace? What would make you say, "Wow"?

5. **Free Time and Possessions:** You deserve to enjoy the fun things of life and have the things you want—including ample time off. This category is about having a quality life—doing things and having things that you really enjoy, like adventure, cool "toys", and hobbies.

In the downloadable workbook which accompanies this book, you can write out your desires and dreams in each of these life areas. You can also write them in a journal if you have one. A huge benefit of creating your Life Vision on paper is that you have an exciting destination that you can regularly focus both your conscious and subconscious mind on achieving.

Get in Touch with Your Big Why

"He who has a 'why' to live for can bear almost any 'how.'"
—*Friedrich Nietzsche*

One of the most powerful and important things you can do as you become a Joyful Achiever is to regularly reflect on and feel the reasons why your dreams, visions, goals, and joy are important to you. This reflection is a key to staying motivated over the long term. The big questions are:

- What is it that you are committed to, what are the reasons behind it, and how does that make you feel?
- Who do you have to BE to reach your Big Goals, what does that feel like, and why do you really want to be that person?
- Why do you want to go to the next level now? Feel it!
- What will next level changes give you and why will that be satisfying to you?

Ask yourself, at the core, what is it that you really want? Do you want peace, freedom, love, and joy in the moment or is it more important for you to feel deep pride in and acknowledgement for your external achievements? Do you want to experience the satisfaction of really making a difference in other people's lives? You can want all of these but it's good to know what's most important to you and what motivates you the most.

Suppose you want to accomplish something challenging, like running your first marathon, and a big part of your motivation is wanting the feeling of accomplishment that comes from pushing yourself and succeeding by achieving something big. Feel that 'why' and know that it is the fuel that drives the 'how' and even the 'what'. Your first marathon probably won't get completed without a powerful 'why' in the forefront of your mind and heart.

To accomplish big juicy goals, we need to dig deep into our motivation by remembering our 'why', especially when things get difficult and we need to apply willpower or focus. When you need to get up early in the morning in spite of feeling exhausted, it can make a real difference in your mood, motivation, and action to remember *why* you are getting up—maybe to deliver a fantastic presentation at an important meeting or to do something positive to uplift your soul or tone your body.

You've probably heard the joke about a bacon and egg breakfast: the chicken is involved but the pig is committed. Which level are you at? (Don't worry, you don't have to die to reach your Wow Goal!) The vibration of full-on commitment brings determination, dedication, perseverance, patience, hard work, and focus. Mere involvement in the process lacks true soul power. So, make your Big Why passionate and then fully commit.

Choose and Declare a Wow Goal

Creating an exciting Wow Goal and getting to work on it, even if you just take baby steps, is going to supercharge your reading of this book. It could be your key to becoming more of a Joyful Achiever than you believed you could be. Choose to go after a Wow Goal that you can likely achieve in a year or less and make it your mission. A mission is defined by Merriam-Webster as **an important goal or purpose that is accompanied by strong conviction, a calling, or vocation.** Your Wow Goal will be your focal point for your growth as you read this book. If you are an athlete or want to choose a Wow Goal around health and vitality, your Wow Goal may be an outstanding athletic performance in an event or an inspiring regular routine. For an entrepreneur, your Wow Goal could be doubling the sales of your service or product, or the development of certain marketing skills or objectives. One of my latest Wow Goals was writing an impactful best-selling personal development book!

Make Your Wow Goal Specific and Challenging

So tell me... what is the Wow Goal that you are going to focus on committedly until it is complete within a year or less? And make sure your Wow Goal is a SMART BHAG! What the heck is that, you ask? Well, I'll wager that most of you have heard those two terms repeated and are actually very familiar with them. But let's go over them so that you can put them in the context of this important step.

SMART refers to the way in which and the degree to which a goal is defined. Each letter in SMART stands for an important part of your goal. Here they are:

- **Specific** - Details please.

- **Measurable** - Give me all the exact measurements.

- **Achievable** - Yeah, it's big but I believe I can pull this off somehow....

- **Relevant** - This goal is genuinely important to me; and

- **Time bound** - I have a deadline to get this done.

- **BHAG** refers to the challenging nature of your goal and paints a picture of a formidable opponent:

  - **B** - BIG Is your Wow Goal big enough?

  - **H** - HAIRY Is it "Hairy," not groveling or making excuses about its existence?

  - **A** - AUDACIOUS The goal should get you odd looks that seem to say: You're going to do WHAT?

  - **G** - GOAL Is your Wow Goal like a target, where it's defined "SMARTly" and you can hit the bullseye?

The whole idea is to make your Wow Goal big enough and expansive enough that it will inspire you to create a bigger and more expansive you. As a Joyful Achiever, you want to consistently have an important goal in progress that will help you stretch and grow. So be SMART—and a little hairy—and watch the greatness unfold!

Write Down Your Wow Goal

Now it's time to write out your SMART BHAG Wow Goal. That's a mouthful, right? Your Wow Goal doesn't have to be that complicated but I want you to test it against all the above criteria so it's big, juicy, clear, and achievable. You don't need to list the 'hows' right now. Just get your Wow Goal down on paper—specific, detailed, and awesome. Let's go:

MY WOW GOAL

The exciting target (my Wow Goal) that l am I committed to hitting is: _____

_____

_____

_____

By when: _____

_____

_____

_____

The Compelling Reason I want to accomplish this (My Big Why) is:

_____

_____

_____

_____

I promise to celebrate my little wins and move towards my Wow Goal with joy!

Signed: _____

5 Tips for Pursuing and Achieving Your Wow Goal with More Joy

1. **Decide to make the journey fun.** Part of putting joy into achievement is learning to relax and have fun. As we discuss in depth later in this book, achieving with joy is a choice and it is a decision that you get to make. Progressing towards your Wow Goal doesn't have to feel stressful; it can have an element of excitement and contain more than a few inspiring moments if you look for them. Regardless of the speed of your progress, don't forget to focus on and celebrate your little wins and notice everything you love about working on your Wow Goal—from the fascinating challenges you encounter to the amazing people you meet along the way.

2. **Protect yourself from burnout and keep your energy flow high.** How great would it be if hard work were the only ingredient necessary for success? The truth is, your energy and mental health are just as crucial, and

working to the point of exhaustion on a regular basis is not joyful or fun and can put your body, mind, and goals at risk. Make it a habit to recognize when you need to sleep longer, take a good nap or two, or just shut it down for a while during the workday (even if it's for 10 minutes.). Intend to work with zest!

3. **On the flip side, stop letting yourself off the hook and tap.** Self-care is a good thing but taking breaks and giving in to distractions too frequently (when you know you should be working) can be a form of avoidance and is detrimental to your success. Sometimes the best self-care is to relax for a few minutes then get off the couch and start tapping (Chapter 3 covers everything you need to know about tapping) while thinking about what's stopping you from diving right into your work. Get yourself motivated and in action of your big goals, especially when you are procrastinating by doing less important things and calling it working hard.

4. **Don't freak out, listen to your negativity, and tap on it.** Now that you've got tapping tools on your toolbelt, you don't have to be afraid of negativity anymore! Not your own, not other people's. Critical, negative statements like, "I've never been a very focused person," or "I'm kidding myself, I can't do that!" are perfect tapping material. You don't have to be afraid of that type of negativity; in fact, just let it be and watch it disappear as you tap your way into success. In Chapter 3, you'll learn everything you need to easily win out over any negativity!

5. **Envision your Wow Goal accomplished several times daily.** Reinforcing the achievement of your Wow Goal again and again is an important strategy for joyful success. Think about having accomplished your Wow Goal

and get into the feeling of it. You might want to have a picture that represents the accomplishment of your Wow Goal that you can look at frequently and feel like you've done it. Tap on any feelings that are not in alignment with your achievement of your Wow Goal, even if the feelings are vague or subtle. It's also useful to write out your Wow Goal regularly and to celebrate your daily progress towards it. You got this!

Chapter 3

A - Activate
The Power of Tapping

Tapping: The Power to Accelerate Change

IT IS VERY important to realize that the things that will stop you or slow you down the most from reaching your big goals are internal—limiting beliefs, fears, and doubts. Joyful Achievers know that it pays to be on the lookout for practical tools that will allow them to change themselves from the inside out. While there are many techniques and systems out there that can help you to let go of negative and limiting beliefs, this book will focus on one of the most powerful and underutilized systems of transformation today, Meridian Tapping, more popularly known as just plain tapping. The tapping techniques highlighted in this book are one, the popular meridian tapping system for emotional release known as the Emotional Freedom Techniques (EFT) and two, my version of tapping, which I call Freestyle Tapping. We will examine these techniques in detail in this chapter.

The Roots of Tapping

Tapping on the meridians is based on the theories and practices of traditional Chinese medicine. Meridians are energy pathways that form a network in the body through which Qi (vital energy) flows. On the physical side, blocked Qi causes pain and illness. On the mental side, blocked Qi can cause fear, panic, or worry. In Chinese medicine, the flow of Qi is restored by using pressure, needles, suction, or heat on a number of the hundreds of power points along the meridians. EFT and other transformative tapping protocols are based on tapping on a few major meridian points to restore the flow of Qi, thereby releasing stuck emotions.

EFT is currently the most popular form of tapping. It has its roots not only in Chinese Medicine but also in a process called Thought Field Therapy (TFT). TFT is a meridian tapping protocol created in the 1980's by a psychotherapist named Dr. Roger Callahan. Callahan astonished both himself and the world when he was able to completely cure his patient of a lifetime phobia of swimming in just one session through a simple tapping routine on several meridian points that he had been experimenting with. Callahan went on to create amazingly fast phobia cures and relief from physical pain by developing his TFT technique consisting of meridian tapping sequences. As Callahan spread the word about his miraculous treatments, TFT began to gain popularity in many therapeutic communities in the late 90s and early 2000s.

In the early 1990s, Unity Minister and Stanford educated engineer Gary Craig, who studied extensively with Callahan, created his own extremely popular therapeutic system based on TFT, which he called the Emotional Freedom Techniques (EFT). Craig's EFT process is simpler than TFT and includes several standard tapping sequences (basic and comprehensive) and accompanying self-dialogue which can be used to effectively address a wide range of ailments, pains, and problems. Millions of people have been exposed to EFT techniques over the last 25 years and there has now been extensive research into the effectiveness of EFT. It has been clinically proven that EFT relieves pain, cures acute anxiety issues such as Post Traumatic Stress Disorder (PTSD), and to helps release limiting beliefs.

The good news for you is that by tapping on a number of vital meridian points on your body with your fingertips you can reliably release tension, resistance, and negativity. When you tap on these points while feeling the emotions associated with your problem, pain, or challenge, the tension you have around the issue decreases and you can often release it completely. With this increasing emotional freedom, you are able to experience a significant or complete reduction of previously painful and challenging feelings and sensations. Your motivation, inspiration, and power naturally intensify and allow you to get results that were previously out of your reach. The tapping method that I call Freestyle Tapping is a simplified version of the EFT process and is designed to be uber easy to learn and self-administer effectively.

And that leads to a wonderful fact about tapping: in most cases, you don't need to work with an experienced or certified tapping practitioner for the process to be effective. Books and EFT videos (on Youtube or Facebook) can give you just about everything you need to make tapping work for you on some of your biggest challenges. Of course, tapping is not a substitute for medical treatment or psychiatric care. Use your intuition and common sense to know when a practitioner or a doctor is needed. Tackling severe trauma or PSTD as a beginning tapper might be very problematic and unwise. If you want to go deeper into the tapping process, and perhaps get better results, you might want to work directly with someone who is an expert at tapping.

It's time to get clear on how to tap. If you are just starting the practice, please keep an open mind. Thoughts like, "this is just some woo-woo stuff," or, "I don't think it's working," may come up, especially when you are very new to tapping. That's perfectly okay. Many times, when I first started tapping, I didn't believe it would work. Fortunately, the effectiveness of tapping is not dependent on you or me believing in it. In the very beginning, your progress might feel slow and you might feel a little awkward, but as you practice these techniques, your skills will grow rapidly and amazing results will follow. The tapping process is easy to learn, uncomplicated, and deeply impactful.

Let's Get Our Tap On: EFT and Freestyle Tapping

Perhaps the primary principle of tapping is that you don't have to (and shouldn't) fight against your negative feelings. Instead, the basic practice of tapping focuses on remaining in your present—even if you're swamped with emotions you wish you didn't have, like fear or anger. By tapping on the points while you focus on your negative feelings or unpleasant physical sensations, you'll naturally lower the intensity of your feelings and release your resistance to the underlying problem. When you are able to stop resisting your negative feelings and soothe them with tapping, they will pretty much release, diminish, or vanish all on their own.

This is the perfect time to go through the "basic recipe" of the Emotional Freedom Techniques. You don't need any special tools or materials to get started—just a willingness to give this method a try. There are also a number of excellent resources for learning EFT listed in the appendix that can be accessed on the Internet.

EFT - The Basic Recipe

1. Identify the Issue You Want to Work On

Identify a problem that is bothering you and that you'd like to work on. Please do it right now. The best way to do this for the purposes of this book is to focus on an issue that has been disturbing you emotionally and affecting your performance. Your problem could be physical, mental, or emotional—whatever feels most appropriate to you at this moment.

An example might be that you are worried about your performance in an upcoming work presentation. At the same time, you are also anxious and feeling some fear and uncertainty about the slow development of your career and your income. For the purposes of this exercise, you should focus only on the work presentation for now. Once that is handled you will be able to deal with your longer-term challenge more powerfully. It will serve you to focus on your one issue as we go through the routine. If other things come up in the process, you can work on them after the intensity of your first issue is significantly reduced.

2. Determine Your Initial Intensity Level

Next, rate the emotional intensity of your current issue on a scale of zero to 10, with 10 being the highest and most intense level of upset/pain and zero being no upset or pain at all. Clinically, this rating system is called "Subjective Units of Distress" (SUDs) and using the SUDs rating helps you to clearly see your progress with tapping. Bring up the issue squarely in your mind and body, feel the emotions and/or the pain, and rate it intuitively as it feels in the moment. Don't worry or overthink the number. Don't think about how it felt yesterday, just right now. In the case of the above performance anxiety example, your worry might be an 8 because your fear and anxiety feel major but not as bad as a super intense 10. What is your intensity level regarding your issue now?

3. Use the Set-Up Statement

At the beginning of the tapping sequence, you'll create a set-up statement designed to announce your intention to accept yourself as you are. Your set-up statement will be in this form:

"Even though I have this problem (insert the actual problem), I deeply and completely accept myself."

You say the set-up statement while you continually and firmly tap with the fingers of one hand on the "karate chop" point on the side of your other hand. Repeat the set-up statement three times as you tap. You are acknowledging the problem and your intention to accept yourself in spite of having it. In the case of the upcoming presentation, you would do a karate chop tap and you might say, "Even though I am afraid that I will do a terrible job presenting today and the attendees will judge me, I deeply and completely accept myself." Now tap on your karate chop point and repeat your set-up statement, based upon your issue, three times.

You will probably feel some resistance to affirming self-acceptance when you are experiencing real problems related to your issue. You might ask: How can I accept my feelings of anxiety or rejection, and why should I say 'I'm accepting of myself' with that giant roadblock standing in the way of my goals? You might feel like you are granting permission to your problems instead of fixing them and that's usually not a happy feeling. But remember, that's the beautiful thing about tapping—by actively being with something that is negative or painful about yourself or your situation, you allow your tapping to release the negative energy that has been troubling you. Contrast that with fighting or denying something you dislike about yourself or your life, which mostly serves to prolong your negative feelings and keep problems hanging around. Non-resistance leads to rapid results with tapping.

4. Follow the Basic Tapping Sequence

Once you've initiated your session by repeating the set-up statement three times while tapping on the "karate chop" point on your hand, it's time to gently tap the other EFT meridian points while stating a reminder phrase. The points illustrated in the diagram below can be tapped with the fingertips of one hand or on both sides with two hands in the following order:

- The tip of either eyebrow in the middle
- The bone on the outer side of either or both eyes
- The bone underneath the middle of either or both eyes
- The point in the middle under your nose and above your upper lip
- The middle of the section of your chin (the indent) underneath your bottom lip
- The area an inch under the collar bone on either or both sides of the middle
- A point underneath your arm on either or both sides of your body that falls about three to four inches below your armpit (at the "middle of the bra strap")
- The area on the top of your head.

Tap at least 5-7 times in each of these places, using two or three fingers, usually of your dominant hand if you are tapping with only one hand. You will have completed a round of tapping when you've tapped through points 1 - 8.

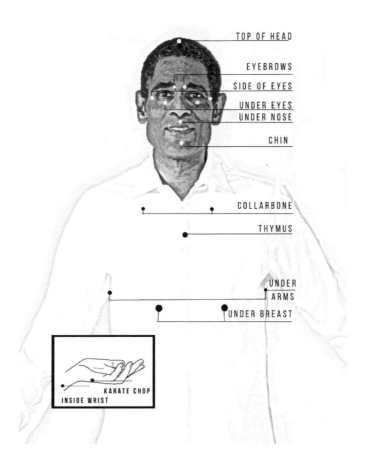

While you move through each of the points, tapping firmly not but sternly, repeat a reminder phrase such as "this problem" or talk about the actual problem out loud to keep you in touch with the emotions surrounding your issue. In the example of your presentation, your reminder phrase might be as simple as "my fear of not remembering what to say", "I'm afraid I'm going to fail", "I'm worried about what my boss will think," or "my performance anxiety is driving me crazy". Your job is to say your reminder phrase(s) again and again as you tap. After you repeat the reminder phrase move to the next point. Give it a try on your issue. Cycle through two (2) rounds of the routine and then relax your tapping and take a couple of deep breaths.

5. Reassess Your Intensity Level

From the time you rated the intensity of your issue at the beginning of your tapping session, has anything changed after your first round or two? Now it's time to re-evaluate. Once more, rate the current intensity level of the emotions surrounding your problem, on a scale of 0 to 10. Based on your new rating, you can decide whether to repeat the process or not. The typical goal is to reduce the intensity level to 2 or below.

Many times, you can bring the intensity level to 0. You can rate yourself after each round or do several rounds in a row before reassessing your intensity level. In our presentation example from above, after going through two rounds of the basic tapping sequence, you may have reduced your intensity to a 5 - feeling that while the presentation is still unsettling, you can handle whatever happens - it will no longer be a disaster that will completely trip you up. And you may want to do two more rounds to reduce the intensity even more.

Where are you with your issue? Did it shift at all?

6. Repeat the Sequence Until You Are Emotionally Free.

At this point, you will want to keep tapping through the basic routine if you are still feeling any negative emotion or pain. Do two more rounds of the basic routine and then take several breaths. Once the intensity reaches below 5 out of 10, you could begin repeating a more positive reminder phrase. Using our example, it could be something like, "I'm open to letting my nervousness go and letting confidence in". After a time tapping like this, you may feel even less hooked and you could add something like: "I choose to feel really relaxed and confident about this meeting". Even if you don't totally feel it yet, you will most likely feel your confidence increase as you keep tapping. My general rule for myself is that if I am not down to a 2 on the scale, I will do another few rounds. You'll most likely be amazed at what you can accomplish within 3-5 minutes of tapping. And, you will find that tapping makes it easier to enter a mode of self-love, acceptance, and joy, even about the previously unacceptable situation or totally stuck feeling that you just couldn't stand when you stated your set-up statement.

There are a number of my favorite tapping tips that are found at the end of this chapter. They will help you be more effective with your tapping. Don't forget to check them out. I've also made a video for those new to tapping that you can find at activateyourgreatness.com/tappingintro

Freestyle Tapping - Tapping… Your Way

Freestyle tapping is basically EFT without the routine. It involves tapping on the same meridian points as EFT, although you might want to add a few more points that I discuss below. The main difference from the EFT basic routine is that with Freestyle Tapping:

1. There is no need to start with the set-up statement.

2. There is no set reminder phrase - talk or remain quiet, the focus is on feeling your emotions

3. You can tap as long as you want on any point - 5 taps, 10 taps, 20 taps or more.

4. You can start with any point and go in a sequence that you enjoy.

5. You can feel free to skip points or add additional meridian points.

6. You are encouraged to do an optional Floor to Ceiling Eye-roll at the end of a round.

With Freestyle Tapping, there is no prescribed routine or formula for your tapping The goal with Freestyle tapping is to enjoy the process of following your intuition and going where your instincts lead you without feeling constricted by a routine. For me, most times I like tapping down the body in a rhythm similar to EFT but instead of starting with the karate chop point, I like to start at the side of both the left and right eye points using both of my hands. But you can do it any way you would like to.

I recommend learning the basic recipe of EFT first and then feel into your preferences from there. You may discover that you prefer a tapping sequence where you skip around a bit, add a few points, or go back to several points. Maybe the set up statement doesn't feel good to you. Maybe you don't want to say something repetitively like you might with EFT—you can just feel into things and say very little as you tap through the points. Or perhaps it feels good to you to be very verbal and ramble about how you feel. Freestyle tapping is all about the emotions and the tapping. It makes tapping on meridian points simple and flexible but no less effective.

With a Freestyle tapping approach, you make an effort to think the thoughts and feel the emotions that you would like to let go of and also feel into any related sensations in the body. You will want to use the same SUDs approach as EFT if it feels helpful to you (as it does to me most times). Suppose you just found out that you lost some money in the stock market and it is going to negatively affect your lifestyle. These worry thoughts could be ringing through your head. You could feel anxious, worried, and frustrated along with some tightness in your chest and maybe a clenched jaw. You could rate yourself as an 8 and start tapping where it felt most needed: first with the basic EFT routine and then focused on a face point or on the karate chop point with an eye-roll or maybe you'll want to settle in on the collarbone point for a good while (20-30 taps) and then move to a long tap on the side of the eye point. Meanwhile, you could be saying everything that comes to mind and expressing the feelings that you think you might be holding in your body. The key with Freestyle tapping is to tap persistently and feel. Bring the issue into the body and mind, let it be and then observe it change as you tap on the points. After you have tapped for a couple of minutes, you should reassess the intensity of both your fear and the tightness in your chest—maybe it's gone down to a 4 or 5. Then go back to tapping and lower the intensity some more. Go ahead and try it on your issue now.

It's great to end your Freestyle tapping session when you feel relaxed about your issue (maybe a 1 or 2 out of 10); you can even keep going until you reach 0 (no reaction or even a positive reaction). When you are at a 1 or a 0, that relaxed, calm state is sure to have you feeling present and engaged—you understand that you have the power to control how you feel even when bad things happen. And that thought feels good!

This is not to say that tapping for 5 or 10 minutes will be an instant cure to all reality-based fears or pain. But there is no doubt that tapping, either with the EFT and/or with the Free-style routine, can help to instill a sense of confidence and control where before there was only fear and worry. Even for the very inexperienced, it can be a calming ritual. Even when you just know the basics, consistent and persistent tapping can substantially release your negative mindset and help you feel like a Joyful Achiever who is prepared to take on any challenge with positivity and relaxed determination.

Achieving Your Wow Goal with the Freestyle Tapping Formula

When we feel stuck and aren't moving towards our big juicy goals as quickly and easily as we want, we can use a simple and powerful tapping formula and watch our feelings change quite rapidly. All you need to do is Identify, Release, and Power Up. Let's go through these three simple steps of the Freestyle Tapping Formula and see how easily we can get into Power Up mode to go after our big juicy goals.

Step 1: Identify (As Best You Can) What's Stopping You

Sometimes it is very clear what is stopping us and other times it seems like the issues are deeply ingrained, under the surface and not as identifiable. While it's not critical to the effectiveness of your tapping, do your best to describe, articulate, feel and maybe even write down what thoughts and feelings seem to be blocking you from your Wow Goal. Start tapping right away, don't wait to figure everything out before you begin because most of the power is in the tapping itself. Sometimes it's even valuable to tap with one hand while you write with the other.

Here are some suggestions as to what might be stopping you or slowing you down from moving ahead with your Wow Goal.

1. You are afraid.

If you feel afraid and the fear is stopping you from taking the required actions, you want to courageously decide to take a small step in the direction of making things happen. Tapping is the perfect tool for turning fear into courage and then moving forward.

2. You don't know what to do.

Many times, things are complex and not at all obvious. You might honestly not know the steps to take. The first thing to do is to tap away the frustration of not knowing what to do and the fear of making mistakes or looking foolish. The next step is to brainstorm your next few steps, not the entire journey. Tap on any fears that arise. When you plan baby steps and start taking them, you gain information that tells you more about the most effective actions you can take to move forward powerfully towards your Wow Goal.

3. You don't believe in yourself.

Many times, this is a big problem. Limiting beliefs in this category usually start with "I can't" or "I'm not". Release tapping will be your focus here—you need to be able to see and feel the possibility of a confident you.

4. You are stopped by the upside of staying where you are.

If we are not doing something that we know we should be doing, the reason is most likely under the hood. Issues in the subconscious, some formed in early childhood or in traumatic situations, can be a powerful deterrent to action even when we have determined our Powerful Why. When we aren't doing something that we want to do, we need to look for potential roadblocks that feel counter-intuitive.

The first is the upside of staying where we are. Often, the urge to stay put and not rock the boat is a major motivating factor in staying stuck. For example, it can be somewhat comfortable to have enough money to get by, but not enough to buy that new car you are lusting after. Even though you want that car really bad and could probably get it if you hustled and put in more hours, you might be stuck, thinking about all the comforts you are enjoying now, no overtime and weekends off, and how you might have to give those up to make more money. You are thinking: "Heck, I'm OK financially, I like my life and I don't want to change. Getting this car is too hard!".

5. You are stopped by the perceived downsides of being successful.

Likewise, there could be voices in your head (or hidden feelings in your gut) telling you that when you are more successful you will be overwhelmed with things to do or that other people could be more critical of you. These and other downsides of success could stop you from fully committing to your Wow Goal, or at least slowing your progress towards it.

This downside pull is most likely under the surface, powerfully working to keep you right where you are. Be on the lookout for these kinds of influences and know that they are roadblocks that you need to guard yourself against. The fact is that it is very difficult to get a Wow Goal accomplished if you feel like you are going to be negatively affected by achieving it. In the "make more so you can get a new car" example above, you might say to yourself: "There's a lot of stress involved with working harder to make more or in finding new ways to generate a higher level of income. I would have to push myself out of my comfort zone and work weekends. I don't think so…"

Step 2: Release Tap - Tap on the Negative

At this point, it is time to start tapping, even though you might only have a basic idea of what is stopping you or slowing you down. Bring all of your fears and worries to the table and verbalize them as you tap. Say the worst things—the things that you don't want, the things that don't represent who you are, but which grab you, even a little, emotionally. The tapping will naturally reduce your level of stress and as you focus on your struggle and tap, the grip your feelings have on you will begin to release. You can feel free to follow a set tapping pattern such as the EFT basic recipe or do Freestyle Tapping. As I do release tapping, I like to go down my body from the head points to the chest area, tapping longer on my favorite points (under the eye and the collar bone points) . The release may take time, so keep tapping as you feel into things. After you have tapped for two rounds, take a deep breath, and reassess things. Repeat if necessary.

Step 3: Power Tap - Affirm Your Success and Work Through the Tailenders

Once your emotions and thoughts have reduced their intensity, it is time to focus on tapping to power up your intentions. One of my favorite ways to move from release tapping to power tapping is with the phrases: "I'm open to", "what if" or "maybe I could". Using these possibility phrases to gently affirm what you want will allow you to release the negative even more and have you naturally feeling what you want to feel. After you feel less weighted by the negative thoughts and feelings (or they are down to 0), power tapping is your key to the next level.

When your tapping has you in a lighter place, it is a good idea to use the first power tapping tool: repeating affirmations that move you closer and closer to your ideal feeling state. Tapping while saying affirmations charges the affirmations and gives them a greater influence on you. The important thing is to just do it—affirm what you want and let the tapping do its work, even if it doesn't feel like it is working like magic at first. The power of affirmation tapping is in repetition over time—keep it up, make it a habit and incorporate it into your daily routine.

The other power tapping tool is to tap while you visualize, which I call visualization tapping. Like all forms of power tapping, visualization tapping comes into play once you have released the majority of your major blocks around going for and achieving what you want. As you keep tapping, you can now let your mind envision what it would be like to accomplish your goal. Bask in seeing and feeling the goal accomplished and bring up happy feelings. Tap and envision your goal like a movie unfolding—seeing yourself hitting your target, celebrating and being grateful. If any tailenders arise, go back to release tapping, feeling your resistance fully and relaxing with the negative voices until they die down.

What are Tailenders?

Tailender is a term coined by Gary Craig to describe what happens when you say an affirmation that is not wholly believable to you at the time. You may have had a recent setback and tapped on it for several rounds of release tapping and now you are feeling better, so you say "I am grateful for this setback" but on the inside your reaction is "I don't feel grateful, I feel mad". Despite your best intentions and expectations, your verbal recitation brings up emotions of anger and frustration. These reactions, at the "tail end" of your attempt to affirm the positive, are called tailenders. We need to pay attention to these reactions and switch our attention back to release tapping on those tailenders before moving ahead with affirmations.

The road to our full joyous tapping power is paved with tailenders. This is not an occasional occurrence in your tapping experience—working with and through tailenders may play a prominent role in your power tapping journey. Embrace your unresolved feelings—there is nothing wrong with them—and as you welcome them and do your release tapping, you give your psyche space to breathe and gradually allow your positive affirmations to actualize in your body and mind.

A Freestyle Tapping Script for Achieving Your Wow Goal

As we have seen in the Freestyle Tapping Formula, there are two distinct parts of the tapping process: Release Tapping (releasing the negative) and Power Tapping (affirming and claiming the positive). Each part of the process is a powerful step towards accomplishing your Wow Goal with joy. Let's dive into a freestyle tapping script that empowers you to achieve big things.

Release Tapping Script: Phrases You Can Use to Begin to Release Your Resistance to Achieving Your Wow Goal

Think of something that you want to do but just don't believe that you can do. Proceed to do EFT or Freestyle tapping while repeating one or more of the following phrases. Alter the phrases to fit your situation. Keep repeating a phrase as you move through the points until you feel that you are ready to move on. Improvise as much as you want to. Let your intuition guide you.

I don't believe I have enough confidence to be the person I want to be.

When I tell myself I can accomplish my goal, I don't believe it.

I don't have the power and fortitude to achieve my goal.

I'm not going to be able to let go of my fear, tension, and stress.

I just don't know how to feel confident and strong about accomplishing my goal.

I don't have what it takes.

When I think of my Wow Goal, I don't feel powerful and confident.

My whole life, I have never been able to accomplish goals like this.

It may be too hard to change my limiting beliefs—why even try?

Deep down, I don't believe in myself.

I am deeply stuck.

And I don't think I can change.

Now, Start a Shift towards Power Tapping

But what if I could change, even a little bit?

What if I could release some of my fear?

What if my fear is not as heavy a burden as I thought?

Do I still need to carry it?

What if I could change my beliefs?

What if I could believe I can make my goal happen?

What if I could relax and open myself to my potential?

What if I could let go of my anxiety?

That would feel so freeing!

I give myself permission to let go of my limiting beliefs.

I know I can release these feelings and these doubts.

Power Tapping Script - I Can Do This

Saying "Yes" to Your Vision, Your Reality, and Your Joy

"Believe that life is worth living and your belief will help create the fact."

—*William James*

I love and accept myself for who I am despite my struggles with my goal.

I am confident in my abilities and skills to achieve what I set my mind to.

I am ready to change my beliefs.

I can reach my goal because I am creative, self-reliant, and industrious.

I deserve to reach my goal and to have all the good things in life.

I am grateful for all the amazing ways that my life supports me to go beyond my old limits.

I do not need to prove myself to anybody—I know I can achieve my goal.

I always find the solution to every problem.

Every problem is a chance for me to grow.

I am not a prisoner to my previous mistakes.

I can choose to be happy even when things are difficult.

No matter what the situation is, I find myself present and engaged.

I am flexible and able to adapt to challenges.

I always expect the best.

I am confident and strong.

My life is beautiful and rewarding.

I am blessed with health, happiness, joy, and abundance.

I appreciate the things I have even as I strive for more.

My mistakes are a stepping-stone to success and accomplishment of my goal.

As I am accomplishing my goal, I am accomplishing my mission in life.

As I move forward, I choose to see the good in others and treat them as if that's all I see.

10 Tips for Getting Awesome Results with Tapping

1. Tap on Both Sides. I think it's best not to get in the habit of tapping on just one side of the body. Mix it up a little, alternating sides within the same session in order to get a full-body experience. I love to use two hands, tapping on both sides of my body at the same time.

2. "Thank You!" Tapping. Tapping is great for releasing your negative feelings, but it can also be an effective method for reinforcing positive feelings—like gratitude! One thing you can do is to make a list of everything you are thankful for. Then read your thank-you list out loud while tapping along. Or you can just say thank you as you are tapping through the points, remembering happy times, and aiming for a feeling of gratitude.

3. Be Creative. It's important to defeat your perfectionist mindset and remember that you can't say the wrong thing while tapping. This is an opportunity to express yourself freely and creatively as you try to resolve your issue. Be expressive and really tap into your feelings. For example, you might want to use metaphors to help really bring out your feelings. You could try something like, "I wish I didn't act like such a mouse when it comes to asserting myself," or, "My anger at Suzy makes me feel like an out-of-control tornado."

4. Argue with Yourself. Sometimes when you are tapping about a problem without a clear or simple solution, you can feel stuck, conflicted, or confused. For example, say you are having a disagreement with your business partner and you aren't quite sure whether the two of you should just go your separate ways or whether you should stick it out. You can see the value in continuing to work together, but part of you feels angry and just wants to burn bridges. One way to deal with this is give voice to both sides of your disagreement as you tap. You don't need to arrive at an answer right away because as you get all of your conflicted feelings out in the open, your intuition will know the best direction to take.

5. Don't Force Change. It is important to remember that the first part of your tapping (release tapping) is all about getting to a place of acceptance then release. It's not necessarily about finding solutions to your problems, although solutions will flow when you get to release the stuck negative parts. As you tap, you want to get to the point where you can love yourself even if you never change. Even if you fail. Even if you can't solve the problem that is haunting you. As you tap, try saying, "I'm never going to stop being angry. And I can handle it!" or "Even if I'm not going to stop hurting anytime soon, that's okay—I'm still alive." Be with yourself as you are and let yourself be truly present in how you feel. Know that however you are feeling right now is not a problem, it's okay; and even if you refuse to change, you know that you don't have to be any other way. **And then watch how things change...**

6. Tap in Public (But Discreetly). Sometimes our strongest feelings arise in the presence of others, but it's not practical and probably inappropriate to carry out a full tapping sequence in front of your boss, or over a politically-charged Thanksgiving dinner. If you're in a difficult or stressful public situation, like a meeting where you're about to make a high-pressure presentation, or you're having a family gathering with relatives you don't get along with, try tapping under the table on your karate-chop point, below your wrist and on right side of your fingers near the nails. Hand and fingertip tapping can be an effective and unobtrusive way to work with your real-time feelings when you need to harness the positive benefits of tapping in public. See the diagram and my bonus video for more information on how to do finger tapping.

7. Add Four More Tapping Points. Once you get the gist of tapping, consider adding these additional meridian points. By adding these points to your tapping routine, you may see even more benefits. They are:

1. The thymus point (an inch above the middle of the chest)

2. The spleen points (the area near the bottom of your ribs below your chest and near the side of the body.)

3. The wrist points (an inch below the crease of your wrist on the inside of the arm)

4. The around the ear points (tap around the ears with cupped hands)

8. Make a Slow Transition from "I Can't" to "I Can." This is going from Release Tapping to Power Tapping. Start your tapping with some version of "I can't do it," and then continue along a progression like the one below. Whether your issue is distraction, pain, lack of confidence, procrastination, or self-sabotage, some variation of the following will enable you to release the issue and then power up your intention:

- I can't do it.
- This is way bigger than I can handle.
- I can't do it now, but maybe someday.
- I might be able to do this.

- Other people have done it, so it's possible.
- What if I could do this?
- It's possible for me.
- I can imagine doing it.
- I believe I can do it.
- I can do it.
- I can't wait to take the next step.

9. Envision Your Ideal Experience. As you focus on creating images and feelings in your mind make them the ideal ones that you really want. For example, say you want to successfully attend a networking event and introduce yourself to ten people, in spite of presently feeling a little unsure of yourself in that situation. Use your Visualization Tapping to go beyond just feeling free of anxiety. Close your eyes and picture yourself feeling truly confident, dressed like a boss, and strolling into the restaurant or hotel conference room with the utmost poise and self-assurance. See yourself walking up to a new networking contact and introducing yourself with a firm handshake and charismatic smile. Imagine yourself building a strong connection and feeling confidence and joy throughout the entire experience. Keep tapping on any tailenders that might show up as you go.

10. Imagine Every Step. As you picture your dreams becoming reality, don't skip any details or steps. Imagine that you are an eight year old child being read a bedtime story. If you skip a page, you are sure to demand, "But what happened in between the part where you met with the millionaire and the part where you closed the deal?" In fact, a 2011 visualization study performed by scientists at Canada's McGill University found that among people who were intent on eating more fruit over a seven day period, the ones who envisioned every step of the process (grasping the fruit, biting into it, and enjoying the taste) were more successful in increasing their fruit intake than those who thought about eating fruit in a more general sense. So practice being as vivid and specific in breaking down your visualizations into steps. And keep tapping as you visualize!

Chapter 4

R - Release the Three Big Limits to High-Level Success

"In the process of letting go you will lose many things from the past, but you will find yourself."

—*Deepak Chopra*

L ET'S CUT TO the bottom line: without a strong mindset and freedom from limiting beliefs, you just are not going to be a Joyful Achiever. You can set big goals, have a powerful why, and even make plans, but you're not getting far if you find that you just can't follow through on your plans, if you constantly tolerate unhealthy habits, or if you constantly give in to other people's requests for your time because you are afraid to stand up for yourself. In this section you are going to dive deep into the power of applying tapping to three major limiting blocks to accomplishing your Wow Goal. To get ready and to practice what we've been learning, take a moment, do some tapping while you think of your Wow Goal and say to yourself (or out loud): "I can do it!" ten times. If that still doesn't feel emotionally right and grounded yet, then say, "What if I really can do it?". Let yourself get into it a bit. This chapter will give you the most value when you intentionally develop a growing sense of certainty and confidence in your ability to accomplish your big juicy goals.

As you now understand, perhaps the main thing that stops us and gets in the way of us achieving our big goals is our limiting beliefs. These are ideas and feelings about ourselves and our abilities, many of which are hidden, which keep us from becoming all that we can be. These beliefs generally relate to our negative thoughts about our ability to accomplish our big goals. These beliefs usually begin with the words: I can't, I don't, or I'm not.

Our task now is to use tapping to identify and release some of these "up until now" limits. I call them "up until now" limits because it is not useful for you to think of your limitations as something that you will carry into the future. By referring to your problems as problems that you have had "up until now", you give your mind the proper framework to work through them, subtly declaring that your limits are retractable or erasable going forward. Next time you are thinking about something that has been limiting you, add "up until now" to the end of the sentence. Make it a habit and see how it affects your view of yourself and others.

Now it is time to go to work on the big three areas of limitation and their associated limiting beliefs. These Big Three are the cause of failure and frustrating results for many would-be Joyful Achievers. They are:

1. Tolerations - I don't like it but I can't do better.

2. Procrastination - I need to put this off.

3. Lack of Confidence - I don't have what it takes to do it.

It is especially important to make significant progress on these three limiters because of their power to be major impediments on the road to joyful achievement. The trick is to catch yourself when you are trapped by one of these limitations and then use the power of tapping to let them go (perhaps again and again).

Stop Tolerating

What is a Toleration?

All of us tolerate, to some degree, things in our lives that we don't like or want. Examples of tolerations include uncontrolled clutter, high credit card debt, constantly saying yes when you mean no, extra body fat, putting up with a tenant who consistently pays late or an employee who consistently comes to work late. Even more, there are all of the things we put up with in intimate and family relationships. There is a big price to pay when we let tolerations pervade our lives. We lower our standards in keeping an undesirable habit or condition around. The things that we tolerate often take up valuable time or space in our lives, drain our energy, steal our peace, and cause distraction. In his book, *The Secret of Being Fiercely Focused,* author Michael Angier states that tolerations can often be the killers of the big three ingredients to success: clarity, concentration, and consistency. You want more of those three, don't you?

Where Are You Tolerating?

The first thing that you want to do is to identify where in your life you are tolerating conditions that you don't want. Take a moment now to identify and write down one or two things you are tolerating in the areas of:

Your Home _____

Your Work _____

Your Lifestyle _____

Your Finances _____

Your Integrity _____

Stop Tolerating Tapping Script

Release the Blocks

Now commit yourself to ridding yourself of these energy drainers—one toleration at a time. Next to each toleration or group of tolerations identify and write down the limiting beliefs that are blocking you. Let's imagine that you have a basement full of stuff that you never use but are storing for a rainy day. Every time you go down to the basement, on some level the mess appals you. Ask yourself: what are the limiting beliefs I'm experiencing? They could be:

1. I don't have the time to clean this up.

2. I have more important things to do than clean up.

3. It's okay, nobody is going to see my mess.

4. I don't have the energy to clean this up.

5. It's not really hurting my life that much.

After you have written down your beliefs, use the script below and start tapping on the first belief of the first toleration on your list. Start by doing release tapping on this belief as you do your best to remember specific incidents and your negative feelings about this toleration. It's important that you let images, feelings, and sensations about your situation come up as you tap. Look for any self-judgment and guilt. Keep going until you have lowered the intensity significantly—go for being a 0 out of 10—unattached and free of all the meaning and judgment that you previously felt about the toleration.

Release Tapping for Tolerations

I'm a failure because...

I don't like how I'm behaving and I'm putting up with it.

I keep doing things that I don't want to do.

I keep tolerating messes in my life.

I keep letting people do things to me that I don't like, and I put up with it.

I keep putting up with things that I shouldn't.

I'm never going to stop doing the things that aren't good for me.

I always let myself get away with less than I am capable of.

I feel guilty because I am avoiding facing my problems.

Affirm and Claim Your Success

Gradually, you want to focus your tapping more and more on the positive. However, focusing on the positive might bring up more negatives (tailenders). Keep rooting out any negativity that comes up by tapping on the resistance and bad feelings that you are experiencing. As you keep releasing your resistance, you will naturally start to focus more and more on solutions and good feelings. Use the power tapping script below and keep tapping through the points until you have a clear feeling of the truth of these affirmations. If some of the more bold affirmations seem like they are too big of an emotional jump, return to starting the affirmation with "I am open to...":

Power Tapping for Eliminating Tolerations

I am open to finding a peaceful place with this toleration.

I am open to letting go of my judgements about having this toleration.

I am open to coming up with a new way to handle this problem.

I am totally willing to take a small step in the direction of getting rid of this toleration.

I feel strong. I know that over time I can get rid of this toleration.

I will eliminate this toleration by (a specific date).

I am committed to living in an inner and outer environment that I love.

I feel so empowered as I eliminate my tolerations.

I am stronger than my tolerations.

I feel grateful that I have the power to let go of things and people I don't need.

I am unstoppable.

Stop Procrastinating

What is Procrastination?

Procrastination is the act of intentionally or habitually putting off important, meaningful tasks. Procrastination is one of the main barriers keeping you from doing the difference-making tasks and moving quickly towards achieving your Wow Goal.

Where Are You Procrastinating?

Almost everyone has a few nagging projects that just never get done. Our rational, forward-thinking minds tell us we should jump right in, but our fears hold us back from ever taking action. Maybe you know you need to start seriously thinking about marketing your consulting services but you have just been hesitating, or maybe you've been avoiding a tough conversation with your spouse about overspending and every time you think about having the conversation, you can't muster the courage to bring it up. Whatever it is, tapping can help us break our habit of avoidance and support us in formulating manageable steps that we will actually take.

To get started, you want to get as specific as you can about the things that you have been avoiding. Don't be alarmed if you have a long list—most of us do, if we are honest with ourselves.

Where am I avoiding doing something I know I should do?

Where have I been putting things off repeatedly because I haven't had time?

Where do I use excuses or just plain neglect to not do things I want to get done?

What is the upside of putting things off that keeps me from taking action?

Let's look at the example about the conversation with your spouse. Maybe you are really angry because your spouse put $500 on your credit card for cool clothes to wear on your up-coming vacation. It's an amount that you really can't comfort-ably afford and is way more than you think is necessary. You found out about this two weeks ago and your anger is still off the charts. You haven't had enough of a rational comfort level to start what could be a difficult conversation. Your vacation is coming up in 10 days and you are worried that the conversation is going to be a disaster and ruin your vacation. You're thinking that maybe if you just avoid this conversation you can have a peaceful and fun vacation. But underneath you know that you are procrastinating on an important task: being in honest and open communication with your partner. Now that you under-stand the 'what' and the 'why' of your procrastination, start tap-ping through all of your emotions: fear, anger, or worry about what could happen until your upset level is zero or near zero. As you tap imagine the conversation happening in a certain loca-tion, maybe having raised voices and heated tones. Keep releas-ing. Keep tapping. As you feel yourself getting freer, let yourself open up to a heartfelt resolution. Maybe see yourself hugging after the conversation. Be mindful to tap on any remaining fear or anger that is in the way of feeling peaceful about the conver-sation. Now you are ready to have that conversation and it will be so much easier on the inside, even if it is still confrontational and argumentative on the outside.

Release the Blocks

It's time to review your procrastination list. At this point, get in touch with all of the reasons and feelings that have caused you to procrastinate on the first item on your list. These may be intense, hard to articulate, and maybe even illogical. Nonetheless, up until now, it's been much more comfortable to procrastinate than to complete the item. With the clarity you have developed through looking at your excuses and justifications, you can now start tapping on all of the stuck spots. Put a number from 1 to 10 on your stuckness and also a number on your desire to put this off. There are probably a number of unpleasant aspects that are keeping you from taking action. You will want to bring them all up as you tap. Find the statements that resonate with you the most and stick with them for a while.

Release Tapping Script for Procrastination

I'm not in the mood to take on that difficult task.

I'll do it later.

I just don't want to do it.

I'm just lazy.

I'm just a coward.

I'll never get it done even if I start, so why bother.

If I try, I'll fail anyway.

I'd much rather avoid this by doing something else that I think is important.

It won't hurt to put it off a little bit longer.

I really don't have time for this.

Maybe I shouldn't take this on anyway.

When I think about working on this project, I feel overwhelmed.

The amount of work this project will require is overwhelming.

Affirm and Claim Your Success

With your resistance significantly reduced after a good tapping session, now it's time to affirm the benefits of taking that action that you have been putting off. By working hard with your release statements, you will have neutralized most, if not all, of the difficult and/or hidden emotions that have been keeping you out of action. Now you can let your tapping gradually guide you to envision yourself taking action and moving things forward. Tap as you say these positive statements several times and feel into your positive future:

Power Tapping Script for Procrastination

I am open to taking action now.

I am open to taking a stand.

I am open to doing the hard thing first.

I can always do one small step at a time.

I am beginning to see how easy and comfortable this could feel.

I am grateful that I have the courage to address this problem.

I am not going to let my fears intimidate me anymore.

I keep going and I learn and grow along the way.

Even though I am not perfect, and a part of me is still scared, I am ready to take consistent small steps that feel appropriate and safe to me.

Remember that this portion of the process does not have to include complete sentences or well thought-out affirmations. It only needs to point to the feelings and images that you want to have happen.

Stop Believing You're Small

Let's face it—a chronic lack of confidence can be crippling.

A lack of confidence means that you don't feel worthy and you don't believe in yourself. Perhaps you are self-critical and you doubt yourself. Some people lack confidence in their personal appearance. Others lack confidence in their ability to voice their opinions. Still others lack confidence in their ability to display excellence, to gain acceptance from others, or to succeed in sports or other endeavors.

Where does a lack of confidence come from?

Lack of confidence can come from childhood. Critical family members and friends can leave a young child uncertain as to their worth and their competence. It can cause a youngster to become self-critical, which can be debilitating and *very* difficult to shake later in life.

Lack of confidence can also come from repeated failure and ongoing self-judgment. It is easy to put ourselves down when we fail, and we can begin to believe that we "are" a failure in a certain area or overall. When this happens, our lack of confidence can expand beyond the few failures to take a more prominent place in our life.

Where are you not believing in yourself?

Lack of self-confidence and low self-esteem are two of the major impediments to reaching your Wow Goal. Are you telling yourself: I can't reach my goal... I can't be that big and bold... I can't have that much power... I can't, I can't, I can't? The biggest contributors to believing you're small are:

- Fear
- Negative self-concept
- What you were told when you were young
- What meaning you've attributed to your failures
- Judgment by others

Take a moment and assess what you are telling yourself that might lead to lower self-esteem. You can write it down for future reference or just stay in touch with it as you tap on the script below.

Build Your Self-Confidence Script

Release the Blocks

Tap as you emphasize the negative and then allow the let-go.

I'm not good enough.

I think there's something wrong with me.

I don't deserve to be successful (fill in what that means for you).

I don't know why, but I feel like at my core, I just don't have what it takes (fill in what means for you).

I'm not lovable.

I'm not that good. Other people are much better than I am (fill in what that means for you).

Other people don't really like me.

I'm not really smart.

I'm not smart enough to be successful.

I'm not attractive enough for a man/woman to want me.

I deserve to be punished for mistakes I've made in my life.

I'm a bad person.

I'm damaged and I'll never be able to heal.

I'm not worthy of love.

I'm not worthy of respect.

I'm not worthy of success.

I deserve to suffer.

I've never been a happy person and I never will be.

I'll never be free from my painful past.

I'll never be able to achieve my goals, so why bother even trying?

I'm damaged goods.

I'm damaged beyond repair.

I'll never be free of the issues that weigh on me.

I'm not cut out to be rich, so there's no point in trying to turn my situation around.

Deep down, I've never felt good about myself, and I believe I never will.

I don't have what it takes to be a happy, successful person.

I just don't have it in me.

What can I do? I'm a born loser.

It sucks big time to be the loser that I am.

I'm always struggling and getting nowhere.

How will anyone like me?

When even I don't like myself?

When even I don't believe in myself?

What's the point of believing in myself?

It's not like I'm going to become more talented, or a different person altogether.

I constantly look for signs of my weakness everywhere inside and outside of myself.

And I see the evidence of my weakness everywhere.

Affirm and Claim Your Success

I am ready for change. I welcome change.

I'm starting to see facets of myself that I didn't know existed.

Maybe I can start to be a little less critical of myself.

I'm open to being a little more forgiving of myself.

Maybe I can start showing a little more compassion for myself.

Maybe I can stop judging myself.

I choose, starting now, to stop believing those useless labels that have held me down.

I am choosing to turn to a new page and write a new story, a story about my success.

I'm starting to feel better about myself, little by little.

And I'm starting to feel good about being me.

My mind is open and free.

I am so grateful for this moment.

I'm feeling calm and confident.

I like myself.

And I'm feeling more and more confident now.

I'm ready to make things happen.

I follow my dreams no matter what.

I can turn things around.

I will turn things around.

I am becoming more and more successful.

I know I can do what I set out to do.

I am determined to do what I set out to do.

I feel much more confident now.

I focus on my growing confidence and it grows even more.

My confidence is growing all the time.

Chapter 5

I - Install Your Joyful Achiever Identity

Decide to be a Joyful Achiever

"A flower blossoms for its own joy."

—*Oscar Wilde*

I HAVE SOME good news: events cannot dictate how you respond to them—you can always choose your response to the events in your life. For some people failure is a stopper while for others, failure is a motivator. It is in the mind of the individual that a response to outer circumstances is born—not in the outside world. Taking full responsibility for your responses is not always easy but the fact is that you always have a choice to empower or disempower yourself when something happens in the outside world.

What this means is that you can choose to be joyful, even in the process of taking on difficult and laborious things. Don't forget to remind yourself of your power to choose. Sometimes it is hard to believe that we have that much choice—that we can actually bring joy to the table when we are tested and stretched. Believing you have the ability to choose your inner reality can lead to dramatically different results in outer reality, according to researchers. A study of over 168,000 students proved that those who believed in a growth mindset (one in which you can improve your abilities by working hard) versus a fixed mindset (one where you can't improve your innate abilities) were more likely to succeed in the long term. When students believed they could get smarter and more skilled by putting in effort, they proved themselves right.

This chapter is about powerfully proving to yourself that you can create a joyful road to success. We are going to focus on "installing" a new identity for yourself, a Joyful Achiever identity, that will make it natural to achieve your Wow Goal. The Joyful Achiever identity is the identity of a person who consistently CAN and WILL enjoy the journey of achievement, a person who is fully committed to success but not attached to the results, someone who handles difficulties powerfully and appreciates themselves and feels grateful regularly. The question now is: How do you go from a "Wanna-Be-but-Can't-Quite-Get-to-Success-Almost-Achiever" or even from a "Rise-and-Grind-Success-Requires-Big-Suffering-Achiever" to being a "I-Can-Make-it-Happen-and-Do-It-Joyfully-Achiever"?

To get beyond these limiting and painful identities, you have to possess three qualities: first, you have to really want to achieve your goal; second, you have to believe that you can achieve it; and third, you have to decide to be joyful as you move towards your goal. A mere "it would be nice to have that big goal and not suffer much" won't be enough to make these things happen. You need to fire up your passion and you also have to believe in yourself. Then you start taking small steps and find ways to applaud your efforts as you go.

Let's briefly review the steps covered in the DARING Success System so far. You first decided on a goal that makes you go "Wow!". Then, you activated your success power through EFT and Freestyle Tapping exercises, releasing your limiting beliefs, and starting to genuinely affirm your success. Now it's time to step into being a Joyful Achiever, appreciating all of your little wins along the way while being committed (but not attached) to achieving your Wow Goal.

When you develop the confidence that you can create joyful inner experiences as you work and focus on doing it consistently, you eventually transform your identity to that of a person who joyfully achieves. Your strategy is simple. Take small forwarding actions with the intention to remain joyful as you take them. It's not necessary to smile as you take huge scary steps —although you can imagine yourself doing that if you want. Reward yourself for taking even the smallest steps by being grateful for even a little forward movement. And forgive yourself when you fall off-course. By building on the little habits and actions, you can slowly but surely create a new emotional identity that can propel you to a state where you consistently achieve with joy!

Once you have made a decision to become a Joyful Achiever, it's time to…..

Choose Three Power Words that Describe Your Best You

An important component of enjoying the journey as you achieve your Wow Goal is to manage your intentions for how you want to feel in your moment to moment experience as you work towards success. High Achievers sometimes overlook the positive emotional part, yet it is so important to you as a Joyful Achiever to pay attention to how you want to feel consistently throughout your day and then make the effort to create the feeling experience that you want.

Let's examine your feeling experience a little more closely. In each moment, there is both your action and the feeling behind your action. Your action is about what you are doing in the moment. Your feelings are about who you are being in the moment. Both are important, and many times we forget that we can and should choose how we want to feel in the moment. It's so easy to believe that how we feel is out of our control and dependent upon outer circumstances. It can certainly feel that way when, for example, you get fired for being repeatedly late or you miss an easy layup at a crucial part of a home game to the dismay of your fans. It's so easy to drop into self-blame and shame in those circumstances, but the reality is that you are 100% responsible for your emotional response to what happens in your life. You can actually be happy and see opportunities when you are fired from a job you hated (even if you were inexcusably late a lot), and you can learn to have a deep forgiveness and love for yourself when you miss an easy shot (even though you lost the game because of it). It's not always easy but the choice is always yours.

What if you made it your mission to be consistently grateful, inspired, and energetic while going after your goals? Would regularly focusing on three power words possibly change the way you feel during the day? Would they change your outlook if you started to believe that you are really in control of how you feel? Right here, right now, is the only time we are actually alive. When we focus on bringing our vitality and love to the present moment, independent of outside circumstances, it can be life changing. We have the power to create joy, forgiveness, and presence even when it's not there in the outside world.

Now choose three power words that express you at your best. Words that you would be proud to have someone say represented you. These are words that you will bring to mind many times a day with the intention of living them. Below are a number of powerful positive words that you can choose from or choose other words that light you up.

Joyful Achiever Qualities

- Focused, Productive, Responsible, Dedicated, Alert, Engaged
- Energized, Passionate, Enthusiastic, Joyful, Excited, Delighted, Victorious
- Composed, Open, Spiritually Connected, Meditative, Calm
- Light-hearted, Mellow, Whimsical, Fun-loving, Humorous
- Inspired, Creative, Curious, Inquisitive, Inventive, Accomplished
- Content, Grateful, Loving, Receptive, Generous, Patient, Worthy
- Compassionate, Understanding, Supportive, Forgiving, Nurturing
- Self-aware, Astute, Observant, Perceptive
- Courageous, Empowered, Confident, Bold, Assertive, Brave, Secure
- Reliable, Honest, Consistent, Steady, Persistent
- Resilient, Resourceful, Versatile, Flexible, Efficient
- Logical, Analytical, Methodical, Wise, Thoughtful

My Three Words are: ——————— , ——————— , ———————

Don't feel stuck with these three words; you can change them anytime you want to.

Your job is to remember these three words regularly. You might want to create a ritual—at certain times (before a meal, when you wake up, before getting into action mode) reflect on your words and how you can embody them fully. Realize that this practice can be life-transforming if you let it. Keep going. You are molding yourself into consistently being your best self.

Here is a short and sweet three-step process that adds tapping to the mix:

Step 1

Freestyle tap for two rounds as you repeat your 3 wonderful words at each point, either silently or aloud. If you find you are way out of alignment with your three words, tap through and release your resistance as best you can.

Step 2

Close your eyes and visualize yourself walking through a doorway into the light of day. As you step through the door, feel light around you as you imagine your wonderful words as feelings in your body.

Step 3

Anchor your wonderful feelings with a Power Move. You might clench your fists with excitement or put your hands on your waist or hoist your hands over your head. Smile and know you've got this, even if you aren't totally there yet! As you keep repeating your Power Move with feeling, you will start to create a stronger connection between the move and the feeling. Over time, just doing the move can produce the feeling!

Be Committed but Non-Attached to Your Big Goals

"Non-attachment allows for full participation in life. It does not mean indifference or carelessness, but rather you should do your best and not worry about the results."

—Zentips.org

Does an emotional attachment to our goals help us to reach them? Many say that you need to have a burning desire and relentless persistence if you want to achieve big things in your life. For some it is unrealistic to think that they could be happy before the goal is reached. However, the concept of non-attachment is key if you want to be joyful as you strive for your big goals. Non-attachment means letting go of outcomes and not tying yourself emotionally to how much you will get done or how it will look. As a Joyful Achiever, you do not let go of your commitment in the name of non-attachment. Instead, you blend commitment with non-attachment to create joyously engaged activity that, in most cases, will move you closer to your goals. Sometimes forgiveness and course correction are needed if you get distracted or interrupted from your important tasks. Just take a deep breath, console yourself for a moment and then get back on track. Your main intention is to focus on doing your best, being present with your task, intending a satisfying output, and being peaceful and accepting even if it doesn't quite turn out as you planned.

Being non-attached is one of the trickier aspects of being a Joyful Achiever. But it is so worth breaking down the inner barriers to feeling unconditional acceptance for ourselves and others and to achieve the peace that it provides. Non-attachment brings your focus powerfully into the present moment—the place that you want to be—and allows you to enjoy yourself with things as they are! When you are not anxious about the future or upset about the past, you have space to enjoy your here and now fully.

Commit to coming back again and again to non-attachment as part of your larger commitment to joyful achievement. It doesn't make you any less effective in going towards your goals, so welcome a little bit of forgiveness and equanimity into your quest, even when it seems like you need a kick in the butt and a talking to. To help you navigate the sometimes-bumpy ride, you can use the following tapping script:

Release Tapping:

At this speed, I'm not going to reach my goals and that's really bad.

I can't let go of this pain of not getting it all done.

I'm not getting enough done.

I should be more productive.

I keep letting myself off the hook.

I don't like myself when I don't do what I say I am going to do.

If I'm not hard on myself, I won't get it done.

I'm not achieving like I should.

I'm not doing the things I should.

I'm just lazy.

I can't accept myself because I'm not trying hard enough.

I can't be happy until things change.

I don't feel good about myself because I'm not getting enough done.

I'm an avoider and I hate that about myself.

I'm too lazy and scared to be a Joyful Achiever.

Maybe I could let go of all these demands I put on myself.

What if I didn't need to push so hard?

Other people keep letting me down.

I can't trust other people.

The people who work for me are lazy.

I need them to do what they said they would.

My team is not working hard enough.

My people are not getting enough done.

I can't be at peace if they aren't doing what they are supposed to.

Power Tapping

I'm becoming more relaxed and in the present moment as I move forward.

I can let go of what I think I need to accomplish and just be.

I can let go of who I think I need to be.

I'm choosing to let go of what I think I need to accomplish.

I'm choosing to let go of who I think I need to be.

I'm choosing to let go of needing others to come through for me.

I can be compassionate and empathetic when people let me down.

I am committed but not attached to my big goals.

I trust that as I keep going for it, great results will be coming.

I see myself relaxed, confident, and not needing external certainty to feel great.

I feel present and satisfied in the moment and allow things to unfold.

I trust that as I relax and open myself to the moment that great things are on their way.

Appreciate and Reward Yourself Frequently

I believe that how you treat yourself as you work towards a Wow Goal can be just as important to your fulfillment as accomplishing the goal itself. And so it will make a tremendous difference if you can learn to celebrate your small wins along the way to success. Celebrate your consistency, acknowledge yourself when you have a tiny breakthrough, give yourself a pat on the back when you start tapping when you need to, jump around when you feel yourself starting to let go of a limiting belief and open yourself up to the joy of the journey.

In addition to celebrating, it's important that you reward yourself, from time to time. It can be anything from taking a little time off, to taking yourself out to dinner, or buying yourself or someone you love a small gift. Celebrating your wins with a reward sends a powerful message to both your body and your mind. The excitement you can generate by celebrating internally and rewarding yourself externally gets your endorphins pumping even more. It sends your mind the message that rewards follow small successes—which in turn, sets yourself up subconsciously for more and more wins.

Another great way to add more joy to the journey is to regularly tap as you think appreciative thoughts about yourself. Use the following script regularly when you want to pat yourself on the back and celebrate a milestone, even if it's a small one. Watch for the tailenders that come up and tap to release them as you move into an appreciative and grateful state of mind.

It's ok to celebrate and appreciate myself.

I can feel good about a lot of things I've done recently.

I like thinking positive things about myself.

I accept myself just the way I am.

I am successful.

I'm good at releasing the negative.

I get into action.

When I see myself doubting myself, I immediately turn it around.

I'm proud of myself.

I love feeling proud of myself.

I'm doing a great job.

How a Joyful Achiever Handles Difficulties Powerfully

When difficult things come up, both externally and internally, it can make a huge difference if you respond powerfully. Difficult people who are frustrating and tormenting us, physical pain, and big setbacks, all happen from time to time. As you install your Joyful Achiever identity you will face your difficult problems in a more relaxed way, perhaps realizing that problems can make you stronger if you let them. Sometimes, if the problem is really bad, you might need to reduce the intensity of your focus on the problem a bit to keep things emotionally manageable. Tapping on the emotions that arise and on the different aspects of the problem will allow you to eventually shift things inside and to act powerfully outside. Here is a tapping script for working on your mind when not-so-good things happen. As you tap on this short script, feel free to add your own twists, turns, and issues that need to be released:

Release Tapping

How am I going to deal with this huge problem?

I made a really bad mistake.

I don't know if I can handle this.

Oh my God, this is really bad.

I can't solve this problem.

This situation is terrible.

I'm totally frustrated and upset that this is happening.

I don't have the resources I need to handle this problem.

Life is hard.

Why is this happening to me?

I'm going to fail.

How am I going to get through this?

Power Tapping

I am open to seeing the positive in this situation.

I wonder if I can turn this around just a little bit.

I wonder if I can accept things the way they are as I do my best to change them.

Even though I have this problem, I refuse to be defeated.

I can relax, trust, and know that my next moves will come to me.

I choose to believe that I can handle difficulties well.

I see this problem as a challenge and I'm up for the challenge.

Time to Turn on Your Joyful Achiever Identity

Take a minute now and imagine going through your days consistently relaxed, energized, and inspired. Imagine really enjoying yourself while focusing on your most important priorities—resting or taking an energizing break when you need to get your energy back. Imagine that you are living as an expression of your three Power Words and finding positivity and enjoyment even as the challenges arise. You realize that with a little determination, it is very possible for you to live with joy on a consistent basis. Now let's bring this vision from imagination into reality. And as usual, we will start by releasing the barriers.

Let's Get Productive

Below are some of the negative beliefs that might be keeping you from being your productive best. It's time to start releasing them from your body and mind. Feel the effect each one has on your body and mind. Then repeat them out loud or to yourself as you tap with the intention to release them from your energy field.

Release Tapping: Let's let go of unproductive, negative attitudes.

I can't do it.

I'm not disciplined.

I can't focus.

I can't get organized.

I'm not good at that.

I'm overwhelmed with everything.

I don't want to.

I'm distracted.

I don't know what I am doing.

It's going to get worse before it gets better.

I have too much to do.

Nothing I do is good enough.

I'm always in my head.

I'm constantly working on low priority stuff.

I hate that even though I am behind, I still watched those tv shows.

I can't stop my bad habits.

I don't really want to stop even though I tell myself I do.

It's really hard to stop bad habits.

Power Tapping: Now that you have reduced or eliminated some of your negative beliefs around your productivity, let's focus on charging up your effectiveness:

I love being productive.

I get things done.

I am focused and productive.

I am organized, efficient, and excellent.

I am a go-getter.

I am increasing my productivity and energy level every day.

I am highly productive and organized.

If I get off course, I keep coming back to my important task.

I love focusing on what's important.

I can get myself to do it even if I don't want to.

I have great habits around productivity.

I can say no to the unimportant.

I love working joyfully.

I am a Joyful Achiever making my big goals come true.

Chapter 6

N - Nail Your Meaningful Action Plan

"Our goals can only be reached through a vehicle of a plan, in which we must fervently believe, and upon which we must vigorously act. There is no other route to success."

—*Pablo Picasso*

U P UNTIL THIS point, we have been talking a lot about clarity, mindset, and empowering ourselves. This high-level stuff, getting clear on your goals, releasing limiting beliefs, and upleveling your mindset turns out to be mostly a waste of time without Meaningful Action. Now is the time to get granular—to talk planning, action, and results. But remember, even as you work like heck on getting your Wow Goal accomplished, the idea is not to think that when you reach the finish line that you've made it. The most important thing to the Joyful Achiever is who you are becoming, not just what you are able to accomplish. After making your Wow Goal (or even bigger goals) a reality, you're going to want to keep growing both as a person and as a professional. You'll want to keep reaching for new Wow Goals and expanding your Life Vision. And hopefully you'll make this ongoing process of achieving your big goals joyful, fun, and exciting. And if not, you always have tapping to help you turn your journey from sour to sweet anytime.

So, let's get started. Your next step is to:

Start Taking Meaningful Action

Meaningful Action, as I am using the term here, is about figuring out what are the actions that are going to make a real difference to your Wow Goal. If you want to be most effective when the rubber meets the road, you're going to want to step back and decide to devote your time to Meaningful Action. Anyone can take action—we all are doing something everyday—but the most successful among us focus on the actions that are needle movers and they move ahead much more quickly. So, let's start to differentiate meaningful actions from the rest and then put them on our calendar. The real question is: Are you ready to go faster?

What Meaningful Action Isn't

Meaningful Action isn't about being busy. It's about getting clear on what will get you to where you want to go with the greatest velocity. Meaningful Action is not about acting fast and furiously because you are a grinder. Meaningful Action is about figuring out what is really going to make a difference and then start taking those actions with a Joyful Achiever focus— engaged, inspired, and non-attached. Meaningful Action is not about handling every part of the job yourself. It's about determining what you are best at and what most needs to be done and then delegating, if possible, anything that is not the best use of your time. Meaningful Action is not about looking good to others by doing high visibility tasks that shine the spotlight on you. It's much more about focusing on making important progress on your Wow Goal and being emotionally in touch with your Big Why. Meaningful Action is about increasing the Wow!

Make a MAP (Meaningful Action Plan)

Brainstorm, Organize, and Prioritize

"It takes as much energy to wish as it does to plan."
—*Eleanor Roosevelt*

I recommend creating a written Meaningful Action Plan for your Wow Goal. It can begin with a simple outline of the various aspects of the goal. For example, in writing this book, the basic outline might include the following aspects:

1. Brainstorming the main message of the book

2. Drafting and editing the book

3. Designing the book cover and inside layout

4. Researching publishers or how to self-publish

5. Launching the book

It is best if your outline is relatively general in the beginning since micro-planning too early can often be counterproductive. For now, just break down your Wow Goal into phases and obvious action steps.

After you have identified the aspects, put on your thinking cap, and brainstorm your Wow Goal. Start listing all the things that you can think of that would take you closer to your Wow Goal and write them into your outline. Make sure to also include the people and the resources that might be involved. This is not the time for accuracy. Just let ideas flow and write them down—sorting will come later. After you have brainstormed for a while, do some organizing and prioritizing of the ideas and actions that you have come up with. Begin to identify the meaningful actions that will make the most difference. Write down how long each action might take.

Put Your Action Steps on the Calendar

Now that you've clarified what you want to achieve and prioritize, you'll need to decide when and where you're going to go about achieving it. Will you work on your Wow Goal for an hour every day? Or will you become a weekend warrior and devote every Saturday and Sunday to bringing your goal to fruition?

At the planning stage, it's important to schedule consistent effort into your calendar, rather than simply assume you'll find the time to make your goal happen. That's because goals are fragile in the beginning, like the first stage of building a fire. It's easy for the strong winds of other responsibilities and demands to blow your match out before the fire gets going. To keep yourself on track, you need to be fierce about your Wow Goal, and do whatever it takes to nurture and protect it. If you have to add a calendar reminder with an alarm to your phone every single day until it becomes a habit, make sure to do so. If you have to tell everyone you know that you can't make any out of town plans for the next three months, do that too.

It will become easier to carve out time in your day for your Wow Goal as your scheduled blocks of focus become a habit. Over time, you'll find your groove easily, and putting in the effort to achieve your Wow Goal will become a regular, established part of your life.

Track Key Measures and Review Your Action Steps

Let's imagine that you set a powerful Wow Goal of making six figures as your own boss in a business that you love. You joyfully see yourself having your own financially successful, impactful, and heart-satisfying business. But you also realize that starting a passion-based business can be a big risk. Time can pass in a flash, without solid financial results. You could easily get financially strapped, start to get down on yourself, and feel that you might want to give up on your business idea.

To keep moving forward joyfully, it will be of great help to keep your focus on maximizing your output of meaningful work. In order to make the most of your days, implement a regular review of your key measures of progress. Determine what daily, weekly, or monthly results are most meaningful to you at this stage. If you're working on a time-consuming project that is hard to fit into your schedule, track the hours you spent working on the project. If you're trying to expand your client base, measure your number of outreach attempts and how many were successful. Measuring and tracking your progress, especially related to meaningful action, can help you make smart decisions from the outset. Plus, you'll start acquiring the essential information you need to adjust your plan for the long term.

Here are some other examples of key measures. What measures of Meaningful Action might be most useful for you to focus on relating to your Wow Goal?

- Number of 30-50 minute blocks per day of uninterrupted quality work on important projects
- Number of words/pages/chapters written per day
- Number of steps walked/miles ran per day
- Number of family dinners per week
- Number of days per week where the internet is shut down at least an hour before bed
- Amount of time per day of quality time with your kids or spouse
- Time spent meditating per day (and resulting mood)
- Hours of sleep per night
- Weight (aim for weekly weigh-ins)
- Savings per week toward a financial goal
- Daily joy on a scale of 1 to 10

If you want to track your progress on meaningful action using an app, there are several options including Coach.me, Momentum, or Habit List. Find the one that works for you and use it daily. A word of warning: the idea is not to let numbers run your life, but to enhance your capability, self-awareness, and joy. Celebrate all the small wins surrounding your progress. And tap to release any self-judgment or comparison with others.

Release and Power Tapping for Brainstorming, Organizing, and Tracking

As you begin the planning process, you may notice that you are not 100% aligned with your planning system. You might want to do some release tapping as you explore your thoughts about planning.

This is not going to make a difference.

I'm disorganized.

Even if I put it on the calendar, I won't do it.

All this planning and I'm still not taking action.

It's hard to come up with a good plan.

Planning has never worked for me.

I'm not a good planner.

I'm not good at tracking.

I don't like tracking and I'm not going to do it.

I'm not doing enough.

I should be getting more results.

I'm embarrassed by my numbers.

I don't want anyone to see my results.

When you are ready, switch to Power Tapping:

I choose to be a little more organized.

I can get slightly better at planning.

I love seeing my calendar with important stuff on it.

I'm ready to focus on results.

I let ideas come to me and I write them down when they do.

I know I can improve and I let go of judging myself.

It's easy to take baby steps and I take them.

Working Meaningfully - The Joyful Focus Routine

Having organized your plan and prepared yourself mentally, now you are ready to make some joyful progress on your Wow Goal—to take focused action in a systematic way while enjoying it all. Wouldn't it be nice to create a time block that is energetically strong, focused, and joyful? Well I have good news—there's a routine for that! It's called the Joyful Focus Routine and it is an important part of the DARING Success System. By using the Joyful Focus Routine on a regular basis, you will have a solid way to gain momentum on your Wow Goal. Do this routine in order to better focus on your meaningful actions—please don't do this routine in order to focus on that 4th episode you are binge watching on Netflix! The Joyful Focus Routine is meant to be done regularly but you don't have to do it perfectly and even if you do just a part or two of the routine it can make a difference. Hopefully, you will turn it into a habit, making sure to do it when you want to make solid progress on one of your important goals.

You decide the length of the routine based on how much time you have, how you feel energetically, and the intensity of your need to get something focused done. I would recommend not doing more than an hour without a break, but you can be the judge of that. Usually a 25 to 50 minute time block with a five to ten minute break will work powerfully. Once you've mastered the steps, the preparation for the focus part of the routine won't take more than 2 or 3 minutes (or maybe 5 minutes if you tap a lot), and it provides powerful motivation for achieving great results during your time block. Let's explore the steps:

1. Set aside your desired block of time in an appropriate place for a period of solid focus on your Wow Goal.

Once you choose the length of time that you want to focus, set a timer. Settle into a place that is free from distractions and then firmly decide that this is going to be a time of uninterrupted focus for you.

2. Turn off the ringer on your phone and stay away from email, social media, and other possible disturbances.

Tell you friends, family or co-workers that you are about to go into joyful focus mode (or just tell them that you are going to be focusing) for your chosen period of time and that you need to not be interrupted.

3. Energetically prepare yourself to crush it (energize yourself).

Do a little light exercise, stretching and/or breathing to get your energy flowing. It can be as simple as a minute jogging in place or bouncing up and down. Have some water or other healthy drink nearby if you can (okay, you can have a cup of coffee!).

4. Repeat your three Power Words at least three times while you tap.

Let the repetition of your power words attune you to the state of mind you are determined to create for yourself right now.

5. Remember and feel your big why for this focused time.

It is always a good time to remember your why and this is a perfect time. Why do you want to be a Joyful Achiever right now? Who or what are you here to serve?

6. Replace any limiting beliefs or mind doodoo with presence and hope (tap for 1-2 minutes).

Do some tapping to let go of any inner disturbances or un-wanted feelings. Get into a place of non-attachment where you are accepting of where you are and open to inspiration and flow. Are you intuiting that your session will be less than awesome? Get to tapping!

7. Resolve to start fast and finish strong.

See yourself on the starting line ready to go. If you like, put on some non-distracting music that can add to your focus.

8. 1,2,3. Go!

It's time to start the timer. Say thank you even before you start for the great job you did preparing. Now...stay put, refocus when distracted, tap again if you need to, and break when your timer goes off. You got this! Great job!

Tap on Your Resistance to Your Meaningful Action Plan

Once your meaningful Action Plan is in place and scheduled, procrastination may raise its ugly head. Ask yourself: When I have clear priorities and a schedule, why might I put things off? Go back and review the chapter on releasing your resistance and tap on procrastination. Now let's look at the best ways to deal with several other issues that may slow you down.

Tapping to Deal Powerfully with Distraction and Delay

What happens if you encounter a few bumps along the way? Let me set the scene for you: imagine you are an executive assistant at a big company working in a cubicle and you want to quit your job and start your own home-based business as a virtual assistant. You dream of spending more time with the kids and less in that crazy traffic but the thought of breaking free of your golden handcuffs and starting a business from scratch sounds scary and difficult! So your plan is to keep your day job to ensure you have a reliable source of income, and commit yourself to working on creating your virtual assistant business as a "side hustle" every evening for a couple of hours after work. At least you'll be making some progress on your ultimate goal of having a successful business of your own.

Imagine that you get working on developing your virtual assistant business by putting in time at night and on the weekend developing your website and your marketing plan. Then an emergency comes up at your job, and you find yourself staying late to fix it. Another day, some great shows on Netflix sidetrack you for most of the evening. On Friday night, you don't say no to friends who want to meet for drinks; after all, your social life is important to your happiness and it is Friday night! Saturday morning, when you had intended to be crushing it, you sleep in and end up spending the morning nursing a hangover. And then there are the kids—yes, they are teenagers but they still have needs you must fulfill, especially on the weekends. After several months of hesitation and procrastination, being your own boss has become a wistful dream.

So, how do you get back on track when, like in the example above, you are being a little self-destructive? One way is to investigate some of the negative beliefs that might be blocking you from moving forward. You might be feeling insecure—your subconscious voices might be bullying you into believing that you don't deserve to achieve your dreams, or that you don't have what it takes to make them come true. You sit quietly and listen as a bunch of negative thoughts surface when you think about your Wow Goal. You realize that you need to free yourself up with some Freestyle Tapping. The following short script is designed to help you prime your mind and body by releasing stuck energy, optimizing your energy flow, and helping you stay positively focused when you get distracted from your Wow Goal. You can tap as long as you like on any of the following script—at this point in your tapping journey, these short scripts are meant to help you develop your own language and style so please add any thoughts or feelings that you need to address to get you back on track.

Release Tapping on Distractions

I'm not on track and I feel horrible.

I'm distracted and I don't like it.

I can't focus on the important stuff.

I never get it right.

I always get distracted.

I can't get back on track.

Why is it so hard to focus?

Power Tapping on Distractions

Even though I'm distracted, I'm ready for a change.

Even though I'm not there yet, I can imagine myself being a focus machine.

I choose to believe in my growing power to focus and not get distracted.

I'm committed to staying focused.

I can and will focus for the next 5 minutes without any distraction.

My focus is growing and it feels great.

I am getting better and better at focusing.

I'm able to focus on the important stuff when I decide to.

Tapping to Deal with Failure and Disappointment in Yourself

This issue is bound to come up quite a bit as you take on big goals and challenges. You are going to make mistakes—you might judge yourself and be massively disappointed with your results. The key to not getting stopped by these issues is to see failure as an opportunity not as a catastrophe. How do you do that? Realize that failure is an opportunity to understand that you are bigger than your results; it's a chance to double down on your determination and release disappointment and frustration. Tapping on these issues will lighten your load and allow you to get back at tackling your Wow Goal with zest.

Up next is a tapping sequence for when you are down on yourself for not getting the results that you wanted. It's intense but by now I hope you know that harsh judgments are acceptable at the beginning part of your tapping script. You want to bring out all the deep unconscious beliefs and attitudes about failure and, quite often, the use of a harsh script will be very helpful to uncover them. You might notice that many of these statements are similar to those in previous scripts. This is because the root of many of our problems and deep beliefs about failure, distraction, and disappointment are similar even in very different situations. As you are clearing your resistance to failure with this script, know that other self-image blocks are being released as well. So, let's go at it:

Release Tapping

I'm a failure.

I can't ever get it right.

I don't want to keep trying, I'll never make this work.

Tapping won't turn this around, I'm hopeless.

I keep failing.

I'm not taking powerful action.

I'm letting my fears get the best of me.

What if I could be neutral about failure?

What if I'm bigger than I know?

What if I'm about to turn this around?

I'm starting to feel just a little less suffocated by this failure.

Maybe things can shift.

I would love to make a shift, even though I'm not sure I believe that I can.

I'm open to considering that repeated tapping might really help.

Power Tapping

I know that I can put the past behind me and look forward with positivity.

I am a winner even though failure is often a part of the journey.

I'm choosing to be above all the negativity.

I see myself getting the important stuff done.

I see myself acting with courage.

I don't need to be perfect, I just need to get to work.

I like to applaud myself for little action, I am proud to be doing this tapping.

Little actions that I can take are starting to reveal themselves.

Wow, I'm turning this around!

I know I'm going to win!

Chapter 7

G - Get Support

"The key is to keep company only with people who uplift you, whose presence calls forth your best."

—*Epictetus*

A N IMPORTANT WAY to make trustworthy progress towards your Wow Goal is by getting support. Keep doing your tapping and create an environment around you that supports you in taking action. In most cases if you are in business for yourself (or want to achieve greater results in whatever you are doing) you'll want to have an accountability buddy, a mastermind group, a coach and/or a mentor (or maybe all four!). This support will allow you to keep moving forward on the road of pursuing your Wow Goal, help you to get back on track when you veer off course and it can even give you new expansive perspectives on getting what you want.

Accountability is often the "get-it-done" factor in life. But once we grow up, we encounter fewer of our friends and colleagues who are naturally willing to push us to the limit and insist that we press on to achieve difficult personal and professional goals. By enrolling an accountability buddy, mastermind partners, or a coach/mentor, you can experience the vitalizing "tough love" you won't get from friends and family. Of course, you might have to release your limiting beliefs in the places you could get stuck around accepting support: the fears, self-doubt, and worries concerning being accountable and being support-able. And as you know by now, tapping will make all that much easier.

First of All: Be Accountable to Yourself

The first person who you must be accountable to is...that's right....you! This basic understanding is the basis of all support that you will receive from the outside. You need to decide that you are committed to pursuing your Wow Goal with gusto and you are not going to be stopped by temporary failure.

There are many ways that you can hold yourself account-able. Here are three really good ones:

1.   Write your promises down, post them in your home and your office, and look at them daily. Block off time on the calendar every day to work on your promised actions and treat that time like an appointment with the mayor.

2.   Announce your intentions to your social circles. Send an email or post an announcement of your promises about getting certain things done. The idea here is to put your-self on the line so that when you make a clear promise, you'll be held responsible for it.

3.   And also don't forget to...

Tap on Your Resistance to Accountability

Sometimes we are afraid of accountability. It can be an invitation to failure if we aren't serious about keeping our word. Plus, there is the possibility of looking bad in the eyes of our friends and family. Accountability takes a bit of courage, especially if what we are promising to do is a little bit of a stretch. But, the upside of being accountable is so important to our progress that we need to just face our fears and push forward on the important things in our lives. So, let's get tapping.

Release Tapping

I don't want to be accountable.

It's too hard to always keep my word.

I don't want to do that stuff and you can't make me.

It's okay to let myself slide once in a while.

Maybe I'm really not serious about this.

Accountability limits my freedom and I don't want that.

I hate being accountable.

I'm afraid I'm going to look bad.

What if I don't make it?

I'm going to fail at being accountable.

Accountability is painful.

I am not good at being accountable.

Power Tapping

What if I could be consistently accountable? How great would that feel?

I'm choosing to be courageous in the face of my fears.

It's ok if I fail but I'm going to give it my very best to keep my promises.

I am serious about making this project happen.

I trust that I can do this.

I'm glad I made this commitment even though it's hard.

I'm going for it!

This project is important to me and I am committed.

I can see myself making this happen, and it feels good.

Get an Accountability Buddy

Many Joyful-Achievers-in-training don't know how to ask for help, even if it would be massively helpful. They assume they should have the willpower, the energy, and the vision to achieve their goals single-handedly. While many Joyful-Achievers-in-training eventually learn how to delegate tasks or outsource processes they don't have time for, these same folks often struggle with getting support for issues like self-doubt or sticking with an important habit. Now that you know tapping, things may be a bit easier, but it still can be hard to admit to others, for example, that your fear of public speaking has kept you from really going for it or that you secretly eat junk food late at night and are carrying around an extra 15 pounds as a result.

But the fact is that reaching out to others for support is an important tool when it comes to staying motivated. Studies have shown that not only do we feel more motivated when we share our goals with other people, but we are more productive when approaching a task or problem with a friend supportively watching. It's been proven that having accountability to a buddy or a group helps us perform better than we do if we just go it alone.

If you're challenged by the thought of doing all that it will take to achieve your Wow Goal, your next step should be to find an Accountability Buddy who can support you and whom you can support. Finding someone who you could tap with would be a big bonus. Make a commitment to each other, like, "I, James, promise to spend half an hour per day writing my book on sales strategies between 7:00 am and 7:30 am", and "I, Brianna, will work on developing my mobile app for three hours every Saturday and Sunday from 10:00 am to 1:00 pm." Then, agree to check in with each other, report your progress, and perhaps arrange a penalty if one of you fails to hold up your end.

Partnering Your Way to Progress: 5 Steps to Joyful Accountability

1. Find a buddy you're willing to commit to. Think carefully about choosing your Accountability Buddy (A.B.). Hopefully, you'll have a fruitful, long-term partnership full of support and "tough love", but this only works if you trust each other, you care about each other's goals, and you're not afraid to call each other out on excuses. It helps to find an A.B. with similar interests and goals to yours, since you'll more easily understand where they are coming from, and vice versa. You get extra credit if you find an A.B. who is also a tapper.

2. Make a regular appointment and stick to it religiously. Having an A.B. helps reinforce the habit you're trying to build as you work toward a big goal. For this to work, you need to meet consistently to check in with each other and report your progress. Set up a regular appointment time, like every Friday afternoon at 5pm, or every morning at 8am, and treat this like an important meeting with a client. If your A.B. cancels more than once or twice in a short span of time or is regularly late, you may need to rethink the partnership.

3. Outline your goals to each other. At the outset of your partnership, you and your A.B. should discuss what you each hope to achieve, and mutually agree on your goals. Break down your commitment into small pieces. For example, if James wants to write a 150-page book on everything he knows about sales, he and his buddy Brianna should decide on reasonable increments for achieving this goal—like completing two pages each day, or writing for a certain amount of time every night. To build a strong habit, it's better to make your commitment as small and regular as possible. For instance, it will probably be much more useful for James to promise to write for thirty minutes a day at a certain time than to just promise to deliver a new chapter to Brianna every week—even if the end result is the same. Finally, it's best to choose one life area (or maybe a couple) to focus on with your buddy at a time. If Brianna commits to doing several things daily to develop a new mobile app she wants to market, it may be too much for her to also be accountable for running five miles a day, reading the news for 15 minutes before bed, and reorganizing her closets for 10 minutes every day after work.

4. Agree on penalties and rewards. To up the stakes, consider making it even more difficult for you and your A.B. to flake out by setting a penalty, and/or a reward. For example, maybe Brianna pays her A.B. $25 every time she fails to put in the promised time on her project. Flaking out will start to become an expensive habit! Equally important is setting rewards. These can be individual (Brianna gets to go on vacation to New Orleans if she sticks to her goal for six months, and James gets to buy that kayak he's been eyeing) or shared rewards, like going out to lunch together to celebrate 30 days of staying on track.

5. Communicate. The most important part of having an Accountability Buddy is leveraging your connectedness to make each other's goals more of a must. That means honestly communicating as opposed to hiding or lying. Discuss with your A.B. what was hard about reaching your goal this week, what went wrong, and how you hope to improve. Don't forget to share your victories both large and small, the strategies that worked for you, and how you felt as you stuck to your commitment. If necessary, you can do this in writing or via recordings but regular live communication is probably going to work best. You and your A.B. should ask each other questions to elicit more insight, plus offer positive reinforcement to rev each other up for the next hurdle. Remember that achieving your goal is more satisfying when you enjoy the process. Even though giving your word and following through can be hard sometimes, working with a partner can step up your shared joy quotient as you both contribute to and celebrate each other's transformation.

Tapping Support for Working with an Accountability Buddy

Release Tapping

My Accountability Buddy is not going to like me, especially when I mess up.

This Accountability Buddy thing will not work for me.

I can't be trusted.

I am going to let my Accountability Buddy down.

I don't want to ask for help.

Having an Accountability Buddy will take up too much time.

My Accountability Buddy is not that committed.

My buddy may reject me.

My buddy may not respect me.

It's hard for me to show up on time.

My partner won't accept me if I am late.

I'm scared to pay a penalty.

I'm afraid I will give my word and I won't keep it.

I don't know if I can be consistent.

Power Tapping

I'm sure there is a way to make this Accountability Buddy thing work and I am going to find it!

I am lucky to have an Accountability Buddy who cares about my success.

I'm not afraid to fail even with someone watching.

I'm determined to succeed and my Accountability Buddy will help me.

I want to have someone to show my commitment to, even if it is a little scary.

The more I give my word, the better I get at it.

I feel empowered by having an Accountability Buddy.

Start or Join a Mastermind Group

A mastermind group is a powerful tool to increase your success. A mastermind is a group of usually five to ten motivated achievers, most often with a similar level of experience or ambition, who get together (either physically or virtually) on a regular basis to support each other in achieving their big goals. Masterminds can serve as a brain trust, accountability partners ,and can provide friendly competition to motivate you to work harder. They can be managed by the mastermind members or run by a coach or consultant. Many mastermind groups meet weekly, bi-weekly or monthly, either in person or virtually and often Accountability Buddies are assigned to make things more personally impactful.

A mastermind usually has a good deal of peer-to-peer mentoring. You can even set up a mastermind to do tapping as part of your regular meetings. As part of a mastermind you will most likely learn a lot of new things, collaborate with other achievers, extend your network, and learn to think bigger. You may be able to join a high-level mastermind if you have the right credentials or you can create a mastermind yourself.

Tapping Support for creating a Mastermind Group

Release Tapping

The group won't like me.

I'm very concerned about my image.

I'm not sure this mastermind is going to make a difference.

I'm not a good leader.

People will judge me for being a bad leader.

I'm not good with details.

I won't be good about keeping time.

I might not like all the people in the group, but I need to pretend I do.

Power Tapping

I am excited about creating a Mastermind Group.

I am willing to learn to be a good leader.

Maybe I can get people to help me with this project.

I choose to focus more on giving than having people like me.

I'm willing to be dependable, even if I can't do it 100%.

I will do my best to make this group valuable for me and for everyone.

Hire a Coach

The coaching process is about working with people to identify the obstacles that are getting in their way, assisting them with finding the motivation to overcome those obstacles, and pinpointing and releasing any resistance to change. A skilled coach can help you transform your career and your personal life into a life that you love. They can help you recognize and utilize your under-used but extraordinary qualities and can assist you in moving along on the path to your highest potential. The best coaches often have you achieve amazing results because they have a hard-won set of skills and qualities. Coaches can serve a critical role that your friends and colleagues can't serve—that of an objective supporter who can help you clarify your goals, identify potential roadblocks, and focus on how to move forward. But what is it actually like to work with a coach? In the context of business and career, coaching is usually a one-on-one relationship formed for the purpose of both professional and personal development. A coach can help you clarify and strategize your business and career development as well as help you strengthen and uplevel your mental and emotional fitness. A coach who coaches you on business success can also help you create a life you love, with an ideal work-life balance, resolution of bad habits and elimination of tolerations in relationships. In fact, according to an article in the Harvard Business Review more than three quarters of coaches who have assisted executives and business owners with business issues also help them with personal issues.

Depending on the arrangement, you and your coach will generally meet one to four times a month to discuss meeting your objectives and removing obstacles to achieving your big goals. A typical coaching relationship lasts between 7 and 12 months, during which you'll focus on the goals you determined at the outset. After reading this book, you might want to look into getting a coach who uses tapping to help you overcome limits.

Tapping Support for Working with a Coach

Release Tapping - Tap on your favorite and your most powerful tapping points, in your own rhythm and sequence, as you say the phrases that bring up negative emotions and resistance for you to release.

I'm not good at being coached.

I don't want to be that vulnerable.

I don't know if I can afford a coach.

I don't want someone looking at me that closely.

I might get a coach and still not be successful.

I might not perform to my coach's standards.

Coaches are expensive.

Power Tapping - Now tap as you focus on the positive, paying attention to any tailenders that need to be released.

What if I don't have to be scared?

What if I am good enough to be coached?

I allow myself to let go of my self-judgment.

I'm even beginning to allow myself to let it be easy.

The truth is that I don't know how good I am until I have finished.

So why should I worry about it when I haven't even started yet?

I will allow myself to just take one small baby step in the direction that my coach asks me.

Nothing big, just one small step, in the right direction.

And I trust that my coach will be happy that I am moving in the right direction.

Coaching is going to work powerfully for me.

I am feeling more and more powerful with coaching.

Why You Might Want to Also Have a Mentor

A mentor is a person who guides a less experienced person by building trust and modeling positive behaviors. The role of an effective mentor is to be authentic, reliable, engaged, and aware of the needs of the mentee. While the coach is not necessarily an expert in the business of the client, the mentor knows the client's business and has achieved much more than the mentee in that field. Whereas a coach can identify the habits, beliefs, and insecurities that are holding you back, a mentor may be able to give you advice on specific issues related to your profession and how to advance powerfully. Some coaches can also serve as mentors—coaches who are experienced in your field can often serve you and your business best.

Finding a mentor could be an important step for some Joyful Achievers. It can also be a humbling move for some, since it involves admitting you don't know some important things, and you need help getting to where you want to be. You need to remember that mentorship is a two-way commitment—you have an important role to play in addition to soaking up knowledge. When you ask a successful figure in your industry to serve as your mentor, it's realistic to assume you are asking an already overscheduled person to make time for you. If they say yes, that should serve as motivation to live up to your end of the arrangement: working as hard as you can to make the best use of your mentor's time, energy, and wisdom. And you in turn, can do everything you can to give back to that mentor.

Release Tapping Script for Mentoring

I can't ask him to mentor me, he's too important.

There's no way she will say yes, so why even try.

I'll be rejected and I'll feel miserable.

I don't have anything to offer them - why would they want to mentor me?

I'm going to let my mentor down.

I don't deserve to have a mentor as powerful as s/he is.

I can't possibly afford a coach mentor.

Even if I pay their fee, I still don't believe I can measure up and succeed.

I'm not ready for huge success so why have a mentor.

Power Tapping Script for Mentoring

I am open to having amazing support from a mentor.

I am open to finding the strength to ask a powerful person to mentor me.

I have more strength in me than I give myself credit for.

I could let myself feel that I deserve a good mentor.

I do deserve a great mentor.

I am getting more and more excited about the possibility of having a great mentor.

I am ready to do great things and I just need proper support.

I am willing to have a mentor inspire me to do great things.

Chapter 8

Conclusion - Your Wow Goal is Calling You

W<small>E HAVE COVERED</small> a lot of terrain over the course of this book, and at this point I want to congratulate you on your staying power. Many who begin a book like this do not get to this point because they get discouraged, lose interest, find another interesting book, or article, or just fail to follow through. But here you are. In this modern day and age, where the attention span of the average person is waning and the level of distraction is increasing, there is a need to make the extra effort to follow through, to return to the task when distracted, and to battle boredom and itchiness with determination. And obviously you are making that effort. Take a moment and appreciate yourself.

Remember Your Why!

It is most often the person with the biggest, clearest, most remembered "why" that remains on the road to reach his or her destination. Really take a moment and congratulate yourself for having a big enough desire for achieving your big goals to get you to this point in this book. One of the ongoing themes of this book is that it is essential to repeatedly think, feel and tap into your Powerful Why for going after your Wow Goal. When stepping up to big goals, quitting in the face of scary challenges and failure can be a very real concern. After all, quitting is easier than mustering up the willpower and determination to push past repeated failures and a lack of belief in yourself. And this is exactly where your Powerful Why comes in... what is it again? Did you write it down? Does it include the Wow feeling of huge success? That's a big reward. Imagining feelings of pride, accomplishment, and mastery can make your hard work and pain feel bearable, especially when it doesn't feel very good in the moment. Your Powerful Why is often the key to bringing the joy. Remind yourself of it often, especially when you feel your motivation lag. And you didn't forget to tap did you?

At a Minimum...

Hopefully by now you have engaged with many of my favorite tools, techniques, and strategies that you can use to reach your big juicy goals while staying energetic and joyful. My intention has been to give you specific and actionable processes to make the journey to your Wow Goal joyful. I realize that there are probably too many ideas in this book to implement all at once, but I hope and pray that you will, at a minimum, tap regularly even if you have to get out of your comfort zone to do it.

Helping my readers to realize and respect the power, flexibility, and ease of tapping is a key reason why I wrote this book. Hopefully, by now, you know that you can use tapping to your advantage just about anytime you need to make a shift in your energy, your mindset, or your strategy. In addition to tapping regularly on your fears and limiting beliefs, please use your tapping powers to feel empowered about your ability to achieve the big juicy goals that make you go Wow!

Let's Recap

Ask yourself now: What key ideas and strategies stood out for me in reading this book and how can I apply them? Too often, a good idea gets the "I already know that" (but haven't applied it) treatment. Then your lack of action keeps that "familiar idea" from becoming an important key that can unlock a new you. Ask yourself: How can I be a more Joyful Achiever and what small step am I willing to commit to making that happen? When I am reading a book like this, I like to write the good and usable ideas down in a journal (or underline them in the book) and then review them several times with a practical implementation intention in mind. I recommend repeating the question: What can I implement and how can I implement it? Let's get more out of our self-development time by being more rigorous in searching for applicability.

I want to leave you with my "at a minimum" advice:

Three Things You Can Implement Immediately

1. **Tap on a Daily Basis** - Start doing it! There is so much ground you can cover just by committing to tapping every day, even if it's just a few minutes. Just ask yourself: What do I want to release now? And then start your release tapping and do a couple of rounds. You got this!

2. **Say Your Three Power Words** - Think of three words that describe the best of you that you would like to carry with you throughout the day. These are words that

make you feel good, even proud! Say them to yourself regularly and watch them bloom.

3. **Regularly Imagine Achieving Your Wow Goal** - Get inspired by something big and juicy and write it down. Get a picture that represents your accomplishing your Wow Goal and keep in a visible place. Know that you are here on the planet for a reason and that reason is to do big, important, and meaningful things. Take time in the morning and/or the evening to do a daily visualization of your Wow Goal. Step into it. Tap on any resistance. Celebrate!

I also created an online workbook and several videos to amplify the learnings that you can receive from this book. Please go to activateyourgreatness.com/joyful to download your free materials.

One Final Tapping Session

And finally, let's end with a Power Tapping round. As you tap, remember to listen for the tailenders and release tap on them:

Even though I am still learning, I am grateful for the power of tapping in my life right now.

I am happy that I am getting better and better at tapping.

With tapping, I can easily release the negative thoughts and feelings that have kept me stuck.

I feel myself shift after I have tapped for a little while.

I remember my three power words many times a day.

I keep bringing my focus back to what I want and what I am grateful for.

I am developing the habits and practices I need to be wildly successful.

I am becoming more of a Joyful Achiever every day.

I enjoy the process of achieving my big juicy goals.

Joyful achieving is becoming more and more natural for me.

I have all the support I need to stay motivated and in action.

I am clear about where I want to go and how great I will feel when I get there.

I am inspired and motivated to take meaningful action towards my big juicy goals.

I love being a Joyful Achiever.

Thank you so much for reading this book. Now that you have at least a basic understanding of the DARING Success System - let's do a final review of the steps you want to take:

1. Decide on a Wow Goal

2. Activate the Power of Tapping

3. Release The Three Big Limits to High-Level Success

4. Install Your Joyful Achiever Identity

5. Nail Your Meaningful Action Plan (MAP)

6. Get Support

Now Go for It. Put the DARING Success System into action and achieve your big juicy goals with joy. May you enjoy a never-ending journey to greater success and fulfillment!

Free Resources For You

Sign up for weekly content and training delivered to your email: www.ActivateYourGreatness.com

Workbook, videos, audio, and other resources for this book: www.ActivateYourGreatness.com/joyful

Facebook Page: @coachjoemitchell

Instagram: @coachjoemitchell

Linkedin: https://www.linkedin.com/in/josephmitchell3/

I would love to hear from you about any questions, comments, successes, or challenges that you may have. Feel free to email me at: coachjoe@activateyourgreatness.com which goes to my business page. I read and respond to all my emails personally. Let's do this! Go out and create some Wow!

About the Author

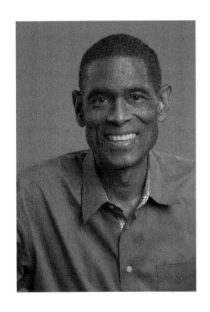

JOE MITCHELL, ESQ. is a High Performance Coach, who has logged over 35 years of in-depth study of personal and spiritual development. Two years after he graduated from Harvard Law School, Joe became a monk and lived in an ashram for 5 years. In his studies over the years, he has done hundreds of self development courses, spiritual retreats, and health related workshops. Coach Joe has been certified as a yoga teacher, meditation teacher, EFT Practitioner and, NLP Practitioner. He is also a graduate of three coaching academies. In 2016, after an over 20 year career as a criminal and personal injury attorney, he decided to turn his heart's passion into a career as a Success Coach, Motivational Speaker and Trainer. For information on Coach Joe's programs, high performance videos and to apply for a Free High Performance Session click the following link http://www.activateyourgreatness.com/free-session.

Made in the USA
Middletown, DE
27 July 2020